SACRAMENTO PUBLIC LIBRARY

D0401893

828 "I" STREET
SACRAMENTO, CA 95814
OCT - - 2003

RUNNER'S
WORLD.
GUIDE TO

RUNNING & PREGNANCY

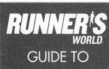

RUNNING & PREGNANCY

HOW TO STAY FIT, KEEP SAFE, AND HAVE A HEALTHY BABY

BY CHRIS LUNDGREN

RODALE

Notice

The information in this book is meant to supplement, not replace, proper exercise training. All forms of exercise pose some inherent risks. The editors and publisher advise readers to take full responsibility for their safety and know their limits. Before practicing the exercises in this book, be sure that your equipment is well-maintained, and do not take risks beyond your level of experience, aptitude, training, and fitness. The exercise and dietary programs in this book are not intended as a substitute for any exercise routine or treatment or dietary regimen that may have been prescribed by your doctor. As with all exercise and dietary programs, you should get your doctor's approval before beginning.

Mention of specific companies, organizations, or authorities in this book does not imply endorsement by the publisher, nor does mention of specific companies, organizations, or authorities imply that they endorse this book.

Internet addresses and telephone numbers given in this book were accurate at the time it went to press.

© 2003 by Chris Lundgren
Photographs © 2003 by Rodale Inc.

All rights reserved. No part of this publication may be reproduced or transmitted in any form or by any means, electronic or mechanical, including photocopying, recording, or any other information storage and retrieval system, without the written permission of the publisher.

Runner's World is a registered trademark of Rodale Inc.

Printed in the United States of America
Rodale Inc. makes every effort to use acid-free ∞, recycled paper ♻.

Photographs by Mitch Mandel/Rodale Images

Interior design by Drew Frantzen

Library of Congress Cataloging-in-Publication Data

Lundgren, Chris.
  Runner's world guide to running and pregnancy : how to stay fit, keep safe, and have a healthy baby / by Chris Lundgren.
       p.   cm.
  Includes index.
  ISBN 1–57954–747–8 paperback
  1. Running for women.   2. Exercise for pregnant women.   I. Title:
Guide to running and pregnancy.   II. Runner's world (Emmaus, Pa. : 1987)
III. Title.
GV1061.L86   2003
796.42'082—dc21   2003010574

Distributed to the book trade by St. Martin's Press

2   4   6   8   10   9   7   5   3   1 paperback

Visit us on the Web at www.runnersworld.com, or call us toll-free at (800) 848-4735.

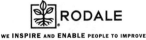

WE **INSPIRE** AND **ENABLE** PEOPLE TO IMPROVE
THEIR LIVES AND THE WORLD AROUND THEM

For Carl, my best friend, soul mate, and husband,
who helped create the subject matter for this project; for
Eric, whose first sentence was "Mommy go running"; and
for Perry, whose solid presence on every run provided
pages and pages of inspiration.

CONTENTS

PART 3: The Second Trimester

PART 4: The Third Trimester

ACKNOWLEDGMENTS

This book wouldn't be a book without the input of many experts. First, thanks to the athletes who shared their prenatal running stories and advice: Kristin Alexander, Shannon Avery, Jill Bagley, Lauri Brockmiller, Karen Cofsky, Lynda Del Missier, Joy Gayter, Wendy Gellert, Kelly Gerlach, Linda Gill, Judy Gower, Susie Graves, Lisa Keller, Laura Kennedy, Diane Krapf, Liz Lincoln, Blythe Marston, Leanne Molinero, Geri Sorenson, Nora Tobin, Mcaire Trapp, and Nanette Zeile.

Special thanks to my friends who granted me interviews and were kind enough to read and critique the manuscript, specifically Melissa David, who provided insight into twin pregnancies and C-sections; Catherine Plichta, who made me laugh until my stretched-out belly ached; and Alden Bumstead, a friend of Catherine's who critiqued my first draft without ever having met me. To Christine Cornell, prenatal water fitness instructor and yet another friend of Catherine's, who answered all my questions on water exercise. To Thelma Robinson, R.N., M.S.N., P.N.P., fellow author, medical expert, and cheerleader for this project.

Thanks to the many fitness, medical, and nutrition experts I consulted, all of whom gave generously of their time: Cindy Bonney, certified nurse-midwife at the Alaska Women's Health Services in Anchorage; Jay Caldwell, M.D., director of the Alaska Sports Medicine Clinic in Anchorage; Nancy Clark, R.D., author of *Nancy Clark's Sports Nutrition Guidebook* and nutrition counselor at SportsMedicine Associates in Brookline, Massachusetts; Geralyn Coopersmith, C.S.C.S., exercise physiologist and owner of Physique Fitness in Ridgefield, Connecticut; James Douglas, M.D., reproductive endocrinologist in Plano, Texas; Elizabeth Joy, M.D., a sports medicine physician and team doctor at the University of Utah in Salt Lake City; Robert E. Keith, R.D., Ph.D., professor of nutrition and food science at Auburn University in Alabama; Debra Kristich-Miskill, certified nurse-midwife at the Anchorage Women's Clinic; Carol Mitchell-Springer, M.D., of the Alaska Women's Health Services in Anchorage; Ingrid Nygaard, M.D., associate professor of obstetrics and gynecology at the University of Iowa; James Pivarnik, Ph.D., professor of kinesiology and osteopathic surgical specialties and director of the Human Energy Research Laboratory at Michigan State University in East Lansing; Sherman Silber, M.D., director of the Infertility Center of St. Louis and author of *How to Get Pregnant with the New Technology*; Judy Van Raalte, Ph.D., professor of psychology at Springfield College in Massachusetts; Frank Webbe, Ph.D., professor of psychology at Florida Institute of Technology in Melbourne and president of the Running Psychologists; Jan Whitefield, M.D., of the Alaska Women's Health Services in Anchorage; and L. A. Wolfe, Ph.D., professor of exercise physiology at the School of Physical Health and Education at Queen's University in Kingston, Ontario.

Special thanks to Patty Kulpa, M.D., sports gynecologist in Gig Harbor, Washington, for granting me numerous interviews; to Joy Backstrum, physical therapist at the Physical Therapy Place in Anchorage, for educating me and demonstrating ways to remain injury-free during pregnancy; and Kathy Hanuschak, R.D., of Allentown, Pennsylvania, for desgining the menus.

To James F. Clapp III, M.D., emeritus professor of reproductive biology at Case Western Reserve University and research professor of obstetrics and gynecology at the University of Vermont College of Medicine, for answering my questions and for his more than two decades of research into exercise and pregnancy. His informative book *Exercising Through Your Pregnancy* gave me the courage to run through my second pregnancy.

Thanks also to Paul Henry Danylewich, director of White Tiger Street Defense in Montreal, Quebec, author of *Fearless: The Complete Personal Safety Guide for Women*; and to Stephanie Shain, dog-bite expert and director of outreach for companion dogs at the Humane Society of the United States in Washington, D.C.

To Linda Honikman of the Road Running Information Center in Santa Barbara, California, for sharing knowledge and providing resources as I wrote the proposal for this book. To Heidi Shelhamer-Felegy at *Runner's World* magazine for providing statistics crucial to getting this project off the ground. To Rodale's Steve Madden, who understood the need for a book on running during pregnancy and worked diligently to make it a reality.

To Leah Flickinger, my creative and diplomatic editor, for sculpting a manuscript into a book. Working with her was a pleasure and a learning experience. To Jane Hahn at *Runner's World* for sharing her expertise in matters of running, pregnancy, and new motherhood. To copy editors Loretta Mowat and Lisa Elwood for their careful attention to details, both big and small.

To agents Janet Rosen and Sheree Bykofsky of Sheree Bykofsky Associates for negotiating my publishing contract.

To my brother Ken Forbes for market research assistance early in the project, and to my sister Anne Wangman (and her sister-in-law Beth Wangman) for helping locate several of the running moms I interviewed. To my mom and dad, Gwen and Lyman Forbes, for raising me to believe I could do anything I put my mind to.

And of course, to Carl for his support, enthusiasm, and many hours of "dad duty," and to Eric and Perry for putting up with a closed door all those days they just wanted to play with Mom.

INTRODUCTION

The seed for this book was planted during the fourth week of my first pregnancy. I wanted something that would tell me it was okay to keep running, that my baby would be fine if I continued the sport I'd pursued my entire adult life. After a desperate and unsuccessful search at the Barnes & Noble near my home in Anchorage, Alaska—the "Pregnancy" shelves, the "Sports" shelves, the "Exercise" shelves—I moved on to the two other major bookstores in town, only to find the same disappointing results.

At my first prenatal checkup, I timidly mentioned my running. "That's fine," the nurse said. "Just keep your heart rate under 140 beats per minute or you could divert oxygen from your womb." I turned green, not from morning sickness, but from the memory of a chest-pounding 8-miler I'd run the night before taking my home pregnancy test. I swore to myself I'd be more careful. During each subsequent run, I'd stop every 3 to 4 minutes and place a finger on my neck to check my pulse. It took little to nudge my heart rate over the limit, so stopping and walking became part of my routine. I began to enjoy my runs less. My frustration grew until I finally quit and replaced running with light workouts on a stairclimbing machine.

My first baby (a boy) was born a healthy 7 pounds 9 ounces and apparently unscathed by my early pregnancy misstep. After confirming my second pregnancy, I shopped again for that elusive book, certain that in the 2 years since my first pregnancy some writer had filled the gap. Again I came away empty-handed—but inspired. The *Runner's World Guide to Running and Pregnancy* had started to germinate. I dug into the piles of research on exercise during pregnancy (and finally learned the truth about heart rate), recorded my experiences in a journal, interviewed medical professionals, and talked with all the moms I could find who had run through their pregnancies.

My second child also was born healthy. Nine months of running had diverted nothing from the womb, which became obvious when the baby emerged at a whopping 8 pounds 10 ounces and sporting an impressive set of lungs that he put to use immediately.

We all have different reasons for wanting to run through pregnancy (you'll find many outlined in the pages that follow). I love the physical and emotional boost I get from running, and I didn't want to let go of that for 9 months. And, like many runners, I thrive on goals. Four weeks postpartum, I began to intersperse some running with walking. Ten months postpartum I ran the marathon I'd fantasized about during my pregnancy. But that's just my story. Pregnancy is a highly individual experience, and your journey through prenatal and postpartum running will likely unfold differently from mine and that of the other runners quoted and profiled in this book. You'll want to listen to your own body and "run your own pregnancy."

Having run all the way through my second pregnancy, I've now answered the burning questions I had when I scoured bookshelves for the volume you now hold in your hands. I've organized the book in a read-as-you-grow format—trying to place answers at the most relevant moments of your pregnancy's progression. Since no two pregnancies are alike, if you don't find what you're looking for in a particular month, read ahead to the next. By the time you finish this book, you'll be armed with the most up-to-date advice from the experts—including exercise physiologists, sports gynecologists, and moms just like you. And you'll have fortified your mind and body for the unique experience of being a runner while becoming a mother.

PART 1:
Gearing Up

CHAPTER 1

ON YOUR MARK, GET SET . . .

PREPARING FOR THE MOST CHALLENGING RACE OF YOUR LIFE

PICTURE THIS: You've just crossed the finish line of a tough race. From the crowd, your husband smiles and waves at you while he holds a small child. The child mouths the word *Mommy*.

Can you see it?

If you're planning a pregnancy, you probably like imagining yourself as a mom. Motherhood can seem like the most normal, mundane thing in the world until you think about undertaking it yourself. Then it becomes personal. And exciting. And scary. All prospective moms-to-be have questions: What will pregnancy feel like? Is childbirth as painful as everyone says? Can I really be someone's mother?

Runners have one more: Is it safe to keep running? Myths about running and pregnancy are common, starting with the notion that you are selfish to even consider it. Here are a few more: You won't be able to get pregnant if you so much as jog around the block. If you do somehow conceive, you'll jiggle that baby right out of the womb. Then your uterus will sag. The list goes on. "A lot of the old docs used to say you couldn't run if you were pregnant," says Patty Kulpa, M.D., a sports gynecologist from Gig Harbor, Washington. "That was the worst advice they could have given women because women would run anyway and just not tell." Dr. Kulpa and other sports-minded medical professionals have dispelled those myths with scientific proof of the benefits and safety of running while pregnant.

For example:

- A 2002 study in the medical journal *Epidemiology* suggests that women who exercise vigorously during a healthy pregnancy can actually decrease the risk of preterm birth.

- According to a 2000 study in *The Journal of Obstetric, Gynecologic and Neonatal Nursing*, participating in prenatal exercise makes women less likely to deliver by cesarean section.

- A 2000 study in *The Journal of Reproductive Medicine* says that exercise lowers blood pressure in pregnant women.

- Exercise can help pregnant women avoid gestational diabetes, according to the March of Dimes Web site. A 1996 article in *The Physician and Sportsmedicine* says that exercise can be part of the therapy for women who develop gestational diabetes.

- An opinion issued by the American College of Obstetricians and Gynecologists in 2002 states that women with uncomplicated pregnancies should get at least 30 minutes of moderate exercise daily.

Babies benefit from prenatal exercise, too. Five years after their birth, the children of exercising mothers scored higher on intelligence tests and had less body fat than children of nonexercising mothers, according to a 1996 study in *The Journal of Pediatrics*. The study's author, James F. Clapp III, M.D., has completed more than two decades of research that shows a positive connection between weight-bearing exercise and pregnancy. (Dr. Clapp has written a book titled *Exercising Through Your Pregnancy*, which discusses his findings and their practical applications to pregnant athletes.)

If you're eyeing the starting line of the great motherhood marathon, here's how to inch forward.

ASSESS YOUR SITUATION

Whether running during pregnancy is right for you depends on your health, fitness level, and pregnancy history. To figure out if you're a good candidate, start by answering these questions.

- Are you a consistent runner? In other words, do you run three or more times a week for at least 20 minutes each time?

- Have you been running for 6 months or more?

- Do you eat a balanced diet that includes all the foods listed in the USDA Food Guide Pyramid—breads, cereals, rice, and pasta; fruits; vegetables; protein from meat, fish, or beans; dairy (or nutritious dairy substitutes); and a healthy amount of fat?

- Do you get a regular period? (This applies to your fertility.)

- Are you willing to be flexible about your workouts?

- Do you have a history of miscarriage (three or more)?

If you answer yes to all but the last question, you're in a good position to continue running through conception and pregnancy. Go ahead and make an appointment with your primary care doctor for a complete pre-pregnancy physical, which will help you rule out any underlying problems or diseases that could make running unsafe for you or the baby later on. Once you're actually pregnant, you will have a different set of circumstances to consider.

If you answered yes to the miscarriage question, you should stop running until you consult with a reproductive endocrinologist or another infertility specialist. She will probably encourage you to undergo testing.

FIND DR. RIGHT

Chances are that you already have an obstetrician-gynecologist or nurse-midwife with whom you're comfortable. If so, make an appointment to discuss your pregnancy plans. If not, ask around. A running buddy might be able to put you in touch with a medical professional who understands the needs of women athletes.

Before you go, determine your fitness goals. Most athletes I interviewed for this book ran during their pregnancies to feel good and maintain a base level of fitness. Some actually tried to improve an aspect of their running, such as flexibility or strength. Most stayed away from speed and distance challenges.

At your consultation, assess whether your doctor will support your running and how well-informed she is about exercise during pregnancy. For starters, does she approve of your running through pregnancy? Can she point you to recent studies on exercise and pregnancy? Has she had other pregnant runners as patients, and if so, what advice did she give them? How does she recommend you measure whether you're running too hard? Many doctors encourage their pregnant patients to run but are not up-to-date on the pertinent medical information. If the doctor focuses on maximum heart rate, she's following outdated guidelines on exercise and pregnancy, and you should consider finding a different doctor. (We'll discuss heart rate and exertion in more detail in chapter 5.)

GET YOUR HEAD IN THE GAME

Your mind is a vital element of preparing to run while pregnant. Get ready to adjust your entire concept of running. You won't be clocking personal records for speed or distance anytime soon. Some suggestions:

Read up. Study everything you can find about pregnancy and exercise. (See the Resource Guide for a list of books, magazines, and Web sites.) The more you know, the more comfortable you'll feel later on.

Interrogate a veteran. Although individual experiences vary, it always helps to hear stories from someone else who's been through it. Do you have a friend or acquaintance who has run through a pregnancy? Talk with her. Ask questions. Chat rooms are another great resource.

Prepare to be flexible. Right now, your greatest concern may be scheduling your runs around your job. When you're pregnant, you'll also have to consider your little rider and the havoc she is wreaking on your body. Learn about what kind of havoc to expect. For example, in early pregnancy, breathlessness can be a problem. Some days you may have to call it quits early because you can't catch your breath. Exhaustion is another common complaint of the newly pregnant. Your daily 6 A.M. run might morph into a 6 P.M. run.

Remember to laugh. A sense of humor goes hand in hand with flexibility. If you can smile at the changes in your life, you'll be happier and willing to be more flexible.

Love your baby. Someday a tiny human will develop right there in your belly. Start to love her and take care of her now by taking care of yourself.

MAKE FOOD WORK FOR YOU

Pregnancy requires you to make good choices about what you eat and drink. That means you should start developing good habits now, especially if you're a junk food addict, so you won't go into shock or withdrawal when you have to do it for real. Begin by adding more fruits, vegetables, dairy, and whole grains to your menu and cutting back on fats. If you're a vegetarian, make sure you're consuming enough vitamin B_{12}, iron, zinc, and calcium. Some more preparation guidelines:

Determine your caloric needs. Your current diet should follow the USDA Food Guide Pyramid and nutritionists generally recommend that active women try to get about 2,000 calories a day. Later, when you're pregnant, simply add 300 calories a day to your normal intake and another 100 calories per mile on days you run.

Concentrate on eating protein and complex carbohydrates. Protein-rich foods like beef, poultry, fish, and beans help build and repair your muscles, and one day they'll help build the baby, too. Complex carbohydrate foods like whole grain bread, pasta, and fruit fuel your runs, replenish your muscles' glycogen stores, and will nourish your baby, who uses glucose as her main source of energy. Without adequate carbs, your blood sugar levels can plummet.

Remember fiber. Running can help keep your bowel functioning smoothly; pregnancy can bring it to a sputtering halt. If you don't already eat 25 grams of fiber each day, begin adding it to your plate little by little so that your body has time to adjust to the increase before you become pregnant.

Drink enough water. Recent studies have called into question the eight-by-eight rule (eight 8-ounce glasses a day) that many of us take for granted. Research shows that you ingest much of the water you need through food and other drinks. Even coffee and tea apparently don't cause the extreme diuretic effect we once thought.

When you're pregnant—particularly as an athlete who sweats regularly—you'll need more fluid than the average person. Among other things, water contributes to the volume of your amniotic fluid, the padding that helps protect your baby. Whether you're pregnant or not, the best indicators of your hydration level are the color and volume of your urine. Drink enough fluids so that your urine is clear instead of yellow and you are urinating every 2 to 4 hours. If you're not used to drinking water regularly, gradually work up to a good hydration level. Accustom yourself to running with a water bottle or hydration system so that you can drink during and immediately after your run.

Take your vitamins. Regardless of where you fall on the dietary spectrum, take a multivitamin every day before you become pregnant. Your doctor can prescribe a prenatal multivitamin or you can take an over-the-counter variety. Either way, it should contain at least 400 micrograms of folic acid to help prevent birth defects. Folic acid is as important to take while you're trying to conceive as it is during pregnancy. Your multivitamin should also furnish you with iron, a mineral that becomes especially important as your blood volume expands during pregnancy.

GET YOUR BODY READY

Experienced runners and some medical professionals make a good case for starting to run well before your pregnancy. "I worry about the woman who thinks, 'I'm pregnant now; I'd better start exercising,'" Dr. Kulpa says. That person could easily confuse running sensations with pregnancy symptoms. For instance, she might mistake the fatigue and breathlessness of early pregnancy for a normal reaction to running. Where an experienced runner would slow down or stop, a novice might think she should keep going. An experienced runner typically knows how her body reacts to anaerobic running (when she is working so hard that her body begins producing energy without using oxygen such as during hill repeats or interval training). In pregnancy, this would be a signal to stop. Novice runners have no such knowledge. To accustom your body to exercise, begin your program at least 6 months before you plan to become pregnant.

To make your adjustment to running while pregnant as smooth as possible, be familiar with your running routes beforehand. Find ones with bathrooms. Look for smooth, flat courses. Evaluate the surfaces you run on. It's easier than ever to get hurt when you run during pregnancy because your joints and ligaments begin loosening in preparation for childbirth. And as your belly grows, your sense of balance may diminish. If you're not already, get used to running on softer surfaces such as dirt roads, smooth and grassy expanses, or cinder trails to cushion your joints. Barring this, gravel is better than asphalt, which is better than concrete—the hardest and worst surface to run on.

Cross-training also can help prevent injury. If you're a one-sport woman, try different types of exercise to find out what else you might like when you're pregnant. One or two lower-impact workouts—such as cycling or stairclimbing—each week will give your heavy body a break, and if you become injured, it won't be so unimaginable to switch to something else while you heal. Chapter 3 describes in detail the many cross-training options available to you.

To prepare your body for the rigors of pregnancy, strengthen the muscles in your torso and pelvic floor, says Geralyn Coopersmith, C.S.C.S., exercise physiologist and owner of Physique Fitness in Ridgefield, Connecticut. The following core torso-strengthening program includes four components: Flexion, rotation, and lateral flexion movements strengthen the abdominal muscles; back extensor movements strengthen the lower back. Unless otherwise noted, these exercises should be performed prior to pregnancy and not past the first trimester, since many involve lying on your back or stomach. Stop the exercises if you feel pain at any time.

Pre-Pregnancy Strengthening Exercises

FLEXION MOVEMENTS

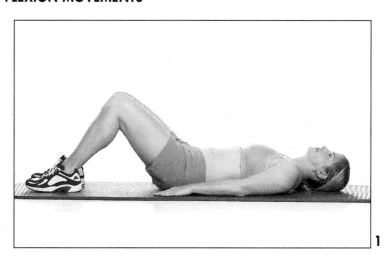

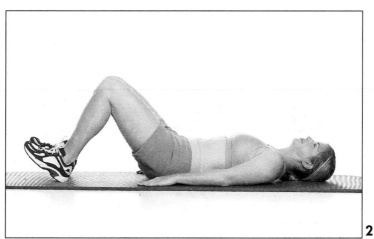

Pelvic Tilt

(1) Lie on your back with your arms by your sides, knees bent, and feet flat on the floor.

(2) Flex your feet, bringing your toes off the floor (to help your pelvis assume a neutral position). Roll your pelvis up and inward a few degrees as you press your lower back to the floor. Hold for a count of two and release. Begin with two sets of 10 repetitions, and work your way up to two sets of 25 repetitions.

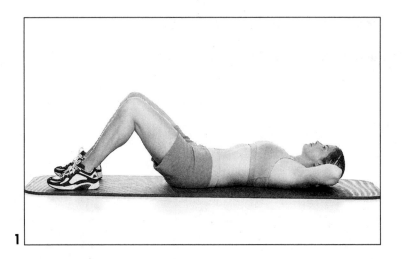

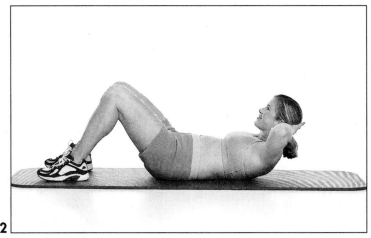

Curl-Up (Partial Situp)

(1) Lie on your back with your feet on the floor about shoulder-width apart. Place your hands behind your head.

(2) Lift with your shoulders (not your elbows) to a 30-degree angle and slowly lower yourself back down. Begin with two sets of 8 repetitions, and work your way up to two sets of 25 repetitions. Don't pull on your head or neck, which will cause neck strain.

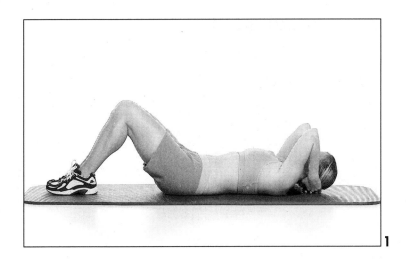

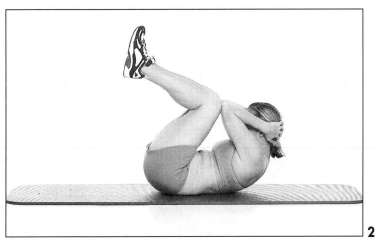

Crunch

(1) Lie on your back with your legs together, knees bent, and feet flat on the floor. Put your hands behind your head, being careful not to pull on your neck during the exercise.

(2) Bring your elbows in close to your head. Lift your shoulders. At the same time, raise your knees so your knees and elbows are touching. Hold for a count of two and release. Begin with two sets of 8 repetitions, and work up to two sets of 20 repetitions.

ROTATION MOVEMENTS

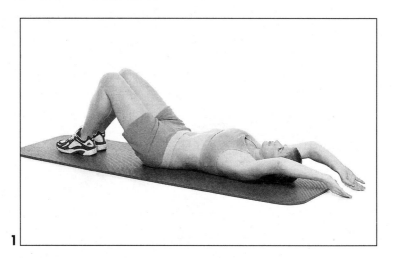

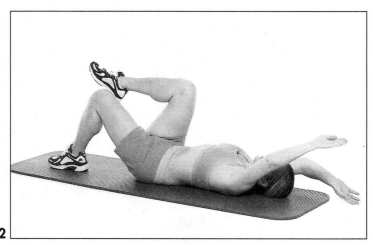

Dead Bug

This exercise will help you learn to stabilize your pelvis. The first time you try it, ask another person to watch you or do it in front of a mirror in case you jiggle unintentionally. (1) Lie on your back with your knees bent, feet flat on the floor, and arms stretched out over your head. Contract your stomach muscles as though you were pulling your belly button into your spine.

(2) Swing your left arm in an arc over your head until it reaches your hip. As you draw your left arm back, bring your right knee toward your torso. Repeat on the other side.

Concentrate on not arching your lower back, pressing your belly button to your spine, and not allowing your hips to shift. Begin with two sets of 10 repetitions, and gradually work up to two sets of 25 repetitions.

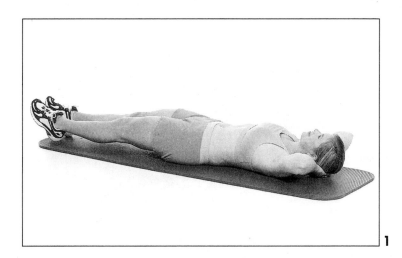

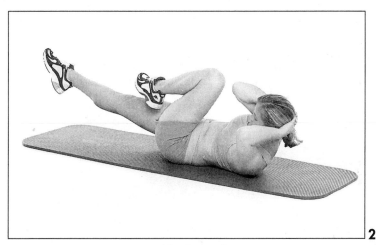

Modified Bicycle

The modified bicycle is a more advanced version of the dead bug. (1) Lie down with your legs out straight, lower back pressed against the floor, and hands behind your head. Bring one knee at a time to a 45-degree angle and begin "pedaling" slowly. The straighter leg will be parallel to the floor, but it will naturally come up a few inches.

(2) Touch your right elbow to your left knee and your left elbow to your right knee. Avoid pulling on your neck. Start with two sets of 10 repetitions, and work up to two sets of 25 repetitions.

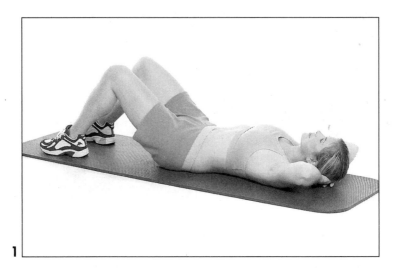

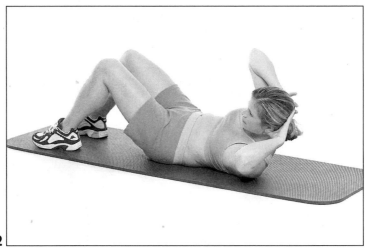

Curl-Up with a Twist

(1) Lie on your back with your knees bent and your feet flat on the floor about shoulder-width apart. Place your hands behind your head.

(2) Leading with your right shoulder (not your elbow), lift your torso and rotate it so that your shoulder approaches your left knee. Slowly let yourself back down and repeat on the other side. Begin with two sets of 8 repetitions, and work your way up to two sets of 25 repetitions. Avoid pulling on your head or neck.

LATERAL FLEXION MOVEMENT

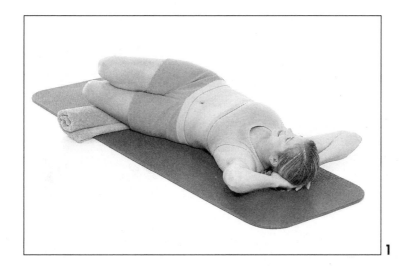

1

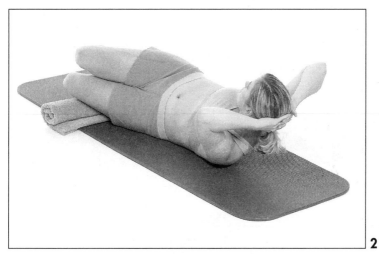

2

Lateral Flexion Crunch

(1) Lie on your back with your hands behind your head. Bend both knees and lower them together to the left so that the left knee rests on the floor with the right one on top of it. (If they do not reach the floor, tuck a small pillow or rolled-up towel underneath your left leg for support.) Keep your left hip against the floor, but allow your right buttock to rise until it is in a comfortable position.

(2) Lift your upper torso toward the ceiling so that your shoulder blades just leave the floor, and come down slowly. Start with two sets of 6 repetitions on each side, and work up to two sets of 12 repetitions on each side.

BACK EXTENSOR MOVEMENTS

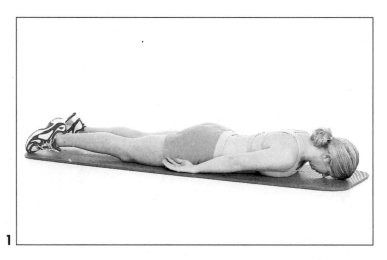

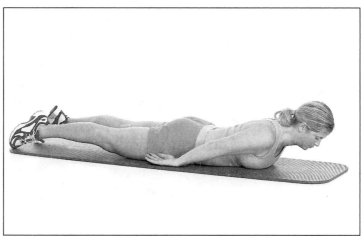

Back Extension

Back extensions are small, gentle lifts. (1) Lie facedown on the floor with your chin tucked in to your chest, resting your arms along your sides.

(2) Contract your legs and buttocks, lift your torso about 2 inches, count to two, and come down slowly. Repeat.

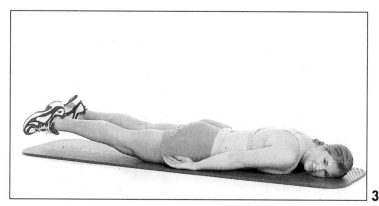

3

(3) Turn your head so that your cheek rests on the floor. Keep your legs hip width apart and lift both legs 2 to 3 inches off the floor, hold for a count of two, and return to the starting position. Do not lift your hips—your pelvis should remain stable on the floor. Aim for 10 repetitions of each part of this exercise.

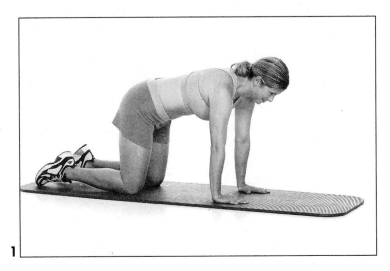

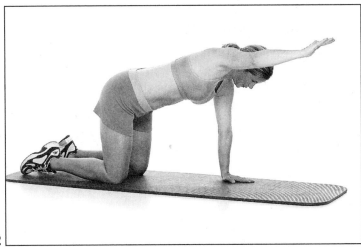

Quadruped

This group of exercises—which also work the back extensor muscles—can be performed during pregnancy, too. (1) Rest on your hands and knees with your head and neck in line with your back. Inhale. As you exhale, imagine drawing your belly button to your spine.

(2) At the same time, reach forward with your right arm so that it forms a straight line with your back, and hold for a count of two. Bring your arm back down and repeat on the other side. To keep yourself in the proper position, imagine that you are balancing a full glass of water on your lower back. When you can complete five repetitions on each side without your muscles shaking and without any pain, you're ready to move on to your legs.

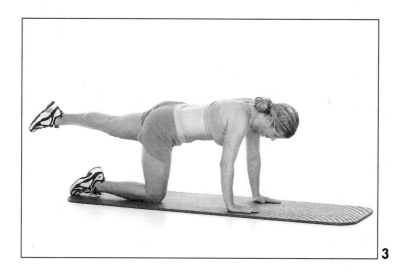

3

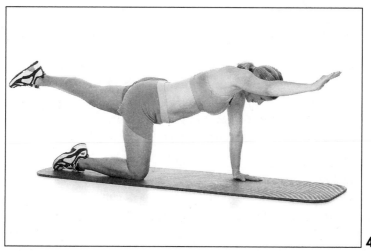

4

(3) Point one leg straight behind you so that it is in line with your back. Hold it still for a count of two and release. Repeat on each side five times.

(4) When you become comfortable with the arm and leg portions of this exercise, combine them to lift one arm along with the opposite leg. Hold for a count of two, and repeat the exercise 10 times on each side. Work up to two sets of 25.

The Three Tenets of
Running through Pregnancy

During pregnancy there are so many things we have to give up: our favorite clothes, a weekend martini, a daily shot of double espresso. Even some herbal teas are off-limits. But if you and your baby are healthy, you don't have to give up running. Here's how to make it through the long haul.

Accept that you're the mom. That means the little person inside you is your first priority, even when she is no bigger than the tip of your shoelace. Run safely, hydrate well, and stay cool. And shelve your competitive urges; you can dust them off later. Be a "mom" to yourself too by staying well-rested and injury-free. Remember that it's easy to become injured when you're pregnant because your joints and ligaments begin loosening early in preparation for childbirth. Twinges of pain should be taken seriously. Your balance may also diminish as you lose sight of your toes.

Remember that pregnancy is not a permanent condition. Envision your pregnant running as a bridge that provides continuity in your life as a runner. Instead of dropping out of the fitness world, you are staying on course; when you reach the other side, you truly will hit the ground running.

Enjoy your running. You're undertaking an entirely new adventure—not a competition, more like a cross-country tour with someone you love. Try not to envy your husband or running group when they train for races you competed in last year. Find new goals, like trying other sports or seeking out scenic routes. Your slower pace and your pregnancy-enhanced sense of smell will allow you to appreciate your surroundings.

Take time to think about the baby, plan for her, and talk to her. You may not be able to keep up with your regular running buddies, so enjoy the little one who comes along for the ride.

Practice Kegel exercises three to four times a week to strengthen your pelvic floor muscles, specifically the pubococcygeal (PC) muscles, which become increasingly important for bladder control during and after pregnancy.

It's easy to isolate your PC muscles. While you're on the toilet, simply stop and then start your urine flow. Contract the PC muscles for 1 second, then release. Concentrate your efforts on the middle section of your vagina rather than the opening. Once you know what these muscles feel like, you should do Kegels when you're not urinating. Hold the contraction for a count of 8 to 10 and repeat 10 times. (For more details on Kegel exercises, see chapter 10.)

Learn to be aware of the transverse abdominus, the deepest layer of abdominal muscle tissue. "It's just a question of teaching a person what to pull in," Coopersmith says. "It's almost like tugging on a very tight pair of jeans, that feeling of pulling in to get those jeans on." By controlling this muscle, you'll learn to keep your pelvis in proper alignment and avoid posture-related aches and pains.

Another posture tip: If you naturally hunch forward, prevent neck and back strain by rotating your chest up and back slightly when you're running (and even when you're not). This will make it easier for you to keep your shoulders, neck, and chin in the correct positions as your belly grows.

CHAPTER 2

THE RACE TO GET PREGNANT

HOW RUNNING AFFECTS FERTILITY

YOU'RE PLANNING TO RUN THROUGH YOUR PREGNANCY, but first you have to get pregnant, right? You may wonder how running will affect your chances of conceiving. The good news is that being fit contributes to your fertility. So does eating well, and since runners tend to choose foods that fuel their bodies, keep digestion operating smoothly, and promote recovery from hard workouts, they often have better diets than nonrunners.

Fertility is an individual matter and dependent on a number of factors—some that involve running and some that don't, some within your control and some outside it. The key is to understand what you can do and be willing to make changes if necessary.

CONCEPTION 101

You've spent years using birth control. Now that you're finally ready to get pregnant, it comes as a surprise when nothing happens. You've always imagined yourself a mom, but here you are month after month with no baby on the way. It doesn't make sense until you understand the basics.

Here's an explanation in the simplest of terms. In order to become pregnant, your ovaries must release a healthy egg that can be fertilized, and your uterus must be ready to accept it. Your brain and body work together to regulate hormones that control each of these dynamics. When the brain or body sends messages of stress, these hormones ebb and flow—and so do your chances of becoming pregnant. Stressors that affect these hormones include too much exercise, decreased nutrition, emotional or mental disturbances, and illness. These stressors interrelate, and even for your doctor or an infertility specialist, it's often impossible to isolate one as the source of your infertility.

The best you can do when trying to conceive is to pay attention to the things under your immediate control: how much you exercise and what you eat.

THE ROLE OF EXERCISE

Your running probably has little effect on your fertility, unless the amount and degree to which you exercise are excessive, says James Douglas, M.D., a reproductive endocrinologist in Plano, Texas. "Excessive" means different things to different people, but most experts agree on one thing: Don't dramatically increase the distance or intensity of your runs when you're trying to conceive. Such changes can send stress signals to your brain

When Is It Time to See an Infertility Specialist?

- If you've had intercourse without birth control for a year, you're under 35, and have regular periods.
- If you've had intercourse without birth control for 6 months, you're at least 35, and have regular periods.
- Within the first 3 months you try to become pregnant if you have irregular periods, no matter what your age.
- If you have miscarried three times in a row.

that stop ovulation or shorten your luteal phase, the stage in which your uterus is ready to accept a fertilized egg. "These conditions decrease the chances of conception and increase miscarriage risk," says Dr. Douglas.

THE ROLE OF BODY FAT

The amount you eat and how much you exercise contribute to the amount of body fat you have. Body fat is measured by body mass index (BMI), which some experts consider a reliable predictor of a woman's fertility. Find yours on the chart on page 28.

With too much or too little body fat, the body loses its ability to activate the hormones necessary for fertility. It turns out that about 6 percent of infertility cases in women result from obesity, defined as a BMI of 30 or higher (although one study reported that even a BMI as low as 27 can lead to infertility). According to the American Society for Reproductive Medicine, excess body fat can cause a woman to produce too much estrogen. As a result, her body will respond as if it's on birth control.

Many women with a BMI below 20 also have trouble conceiving, says Robert E. Keith, R.D., Ph.D., professor of nutrition and food science at Auburn University in Alabama. Other experts draw the line at a BMI as low as 18 or 19. Of course, leanness and fertility aren't mutually exclusive. "Plenty of thin women are perfectly fertile," says Sherman Silber, M.D., author of *How to Get Pregnant with the New Technology* and director of the Infertility Center of St. Louis. "They have regular periods, and when they want to have babies, they're able to."

To maintain a healthy BMI, try to eat about 2,000 calories per day, with 100 additional calories per mile on days you run. For food selection, follow the USDA Food Guide Pyramid, and try to make your calorie breakdown 55 to 60 percent carbohydrates, 25 to 30 percent fat, and 10 to 15 percent protein.

Body Mass Index (BMI)

HEIGHT	WEIGHT (IN POUNDS)													
4'10"	91	96	100	105	110	115	119	124	129	134	138	143	148	153
4'11"	94	99	104	109	114	119	124	128	133	138	143	148	153	158
5'0"	97	102	107	112	118	123	128	133	138	143	148	153	158	163
5'1"	100	106	111	116	122	127	132	137	143	148	153	158	164	169
5'2"	104	109	115	120	126	131	136	142	147	153	158	164	169	174
5'3"	107	113	118	124	130	135	141	146	152	158	163	169	175	180
5'4"	110	116	122	128	134	140	145	151	157	163	169	174	180	186
5'5"	114	120	126	132	138	144	150	156	162	168	174	180	186	192
5'6"	118	124	130	136	142	148	155	161	167	173	179	186	192	198
5'7"	121	127	134	140	146	153	159	166	172	178	185	191	197	204
5'8"	125	131	138	144	151	158	164	171	177	184	190	197	203	210
5'9"	128	135	142	149	155	162	169	176	182	189	196	203	209	216
5'10"	132	139	146	153	160	167	174	181	188	195	202	207	215	222
5'11"	136	143	150	157	165	172	179	186	193	200	208	215	222	229
6'0"	140	147	154	162	169	177	184	191	199	206	213	221	228	235
BMI	19	20	21	22	23	24	25	26	27	28	29	30	31	32

SOURCE: National Heart, Lung, and Blood Institute

EATING DISORDERS AND THEIR CONSEQUENCES

No one knows exactly how many female athletes suffer from eating disorders. Depending on which study you read, the numbers range from 15 to 62 percent. Some experts say runners are less prone to eating disorders than athletes judged on appearance, such as gymnasts and figure skaters. However, the National Collegiate Athletic Association ranked cross-country runners as having the second highest prevalence of eating disorders among college athletes. Since an eating disorder can have a disastrous effect on your fertility—and on the baby's health if you do get pregnant—it's important that you address the issue if you suffer from one.

Athletes with eating disorders consider food as something that slows them down rather than something that provides much-needed energy. "There's a perception, at least amongst sports where being thin and lean confers a competitive advantage, that thinness over everything else wins," says Elizabeth Joy, M.D., a sports medicine physician and team doctor at the University of Utah in Salt Lake City. "It's 'Be thin to win.'"

Eating disorders include:

- **Anorexia nervosa:** Fasting and, in some cases, bingeing and purging and/or excessive exercise. Many anorexics become runners because of the high number of calories they can burn in each workout.

- **Bulimia:** Overeating and purging by vomiting, use of laxatives, or excessive exercise. One form of bulimia is actually called *exercise bulimia.*

- **Calorie restriction:** Eating insufficient calories to cover the body's energy needs, especially when combined with vigorous exercise.

Any of these disorders can cause you to stop ovulating and having periods (called *amenorrhea* in medicalese), which in turn can cause

Enhance Your Chances

If you were preparing for a race, you'd tailor your workouts to achieve the best possible result. Instead of jogging a lap or two around the track and hoping for good luck, you'd schedule speed workouts, tempo runs, long runs, and medium-length runs, and you'd plan to peak at just the right time. Preparing for conception is similar. For maximum success, find out when you ovulate and time intercourse accordingly. Here are a few ways you can do this.

- Purchase an ovulation predictor kit, which is as simple to use as a home pregnancy test. These urine-testing devices monitor the luteinizing hormone in your blood, a substance that surges 12 to 36 hours prior to ovulation. The tests give you an accurate view of your "window of opportunity," but are fairly expensive at around $20 to $40 per cycle.

- Purchase a saliva ovulation detector, which is a mini microscope that reveals changes in the structure of your saliva during your fertile days. This product costs $30 to $60 or more but can be reused many times.

- Observe your cervical mucus, which costs nothing. Your cervix will begin producing mucus a few days after your period ends. The mucus will start out sticky and then thin out, and you will likely notice it on your toilet paper when you go to the bathroom. When the mucus has

bone fractures indicating that you may be developing osteoporosis. Taken together, these three symptoms— disordered eating, amenorrhea, and osteoporosis—form a problem experts call *Female Athlete Triad.*

Female Athlete Triad is a reliable predictor of infertility, mainly because the absence of your periods reveals that you're not ovulating. What does it take to overcome the Triad? While a proper diet is the "cornerstone of treatment," according to Dr. Joy, you really need the expertise of three types of health professionals to beat the problem: a nutritionist to discuss proper diet and eating behaviors, a mental health counselor to help confront the psychological issues that led to the become clear and stretchy, it means you're just about to ovulate or have just ovulated, and this is your checkered flag to begin (or continue) having intercourse. The clear, stretchy type of mucus will last about two days, after which it will thicken up and get sticky again, signaling the end of your fertile phase. Your doctor can help you understand this process in greater detail.

- Take your basal body temperature (BBT) at the same time each morning before you get out of bed. For less than $10, you can buy a kit that includes a BBT thermometer and a chart for tracking your temperature, which rises *after* ovulation. BBT kits won't tell you when to time intercourse the first time around, but they can be useful for future reference. Most experts recommend charting BBT for 3 months to draw a clear picture of your ovulation schedule.

Even if you don't get pregnant right away, each of these methods points to the interval of time during which you ovulate, and you can use the information in subsequent months. Some experts suggest using a combination of methods to get the most comprehensive understanding of your fertility cycle. Ovulation predictor kits, saliva ovulation detectors, and BBT thermometers are available at most drugstores and discount stores, but you can find the best prices through online retailers.

problem in the first place, and a physician to manage the physical symptoms, such as bone-density loss and infertility.

If you suspect you have an eating disorder or Female Athlete Triad, discuss it with your obstetrician, who may offer a referral to an infertility specialist, nutritionist, or other health professional. Pay close attention to the quality and quantity of what you eat, making sure to include hearty helpings of protein and calcium in your diet. "When people are short on calories, they generally need more protein, because protein gets used for fuel instead of being used to protect the muscles," says Nancy Clark, R.D., author of *Nancy Clark's Sports Nutrition Guidebook* and nutrition counselor at SportsMedicine Associates in

De-Stress for Success

Numerous studies point to regular exercise like running as a stress reliever. This is a good thing for fertility, since anxiety can prevent ovulation, says Sherman Silber, M.D., author of *How to Get Pregnant with the New Technology* and director of the Infertility Center of St. Louis. If your running reduces your stress levels, it may contribute to your fertility. Of course, if your running becomes excessive and begins causing anxiety, you'll need to reset your priorities.

Brookline, Massachusetts. "Those calories should come from things like yogurt and low-fat milk, which contain not only protein but the calcium that's important for the bones." Clark also urges athletes recovering from eating disorders to eat "healthy" fats that come from nuts (including peanut butter), salmon, and olive oil.

FERTILITY AND YOUR RUNNING MATE: WHAT HE NEEDS TO KNOW

If your husband also is a runner or another type of athlete, you both may have questions about whether his training affects his fertility. For one thing, men often worry that exercise will cause the temperature of their testicles to rise, thereby compromising sperm production.

Tell your partner to rest easy. In their position outside the body, the testicles adapt to the temperature around them rather than to the body's core temperature, says Dr. Silber. Testicles can produce sperm when their temperature is 94°F or cooler. And during regular exercise, they usually don't go above that threshold (unless a man is severely overheated, nearly to the point of heatstroke). That means your mate doesn't have to refrain from exercise. And you want him to exercise—when men become overweight, their bodies secrete too much estrogen (just like women), which compromises their ability to produce viable sperm.

Your mate does have to stay out of the hot tub, though. "Testicular temperature is strictly dependent upon the temperature of the scrotum," says Dr. Silber. "And the temperature of the scrotum will be the same as the temperature of the water."

Your partner should also eat a healthy diet and avoid dietary supplements other than standard vitamins and multivitamin tablets. Men's sperm counts can suffer from some of the ingredients in dietary supplements, particularly anabolic steroids. One natural (and legal) steroid commonly found in supplements is androstenedione, which gained notoriety during Mark McGwire's 1998 record-shattering home-run race. Studies have shown that androstenedione increases estrogen levels, which harm sperm count. "I've seen a lot of men who think they're taking safe, nonsteroid dietary supplements and their sperm count goes down," Dr. Silber says. "If there's a big claim about the vitamin because it's part of a nutritional [program] designed for body builders and athletes, beware of it."

CHAPTER 3

RUNNING
REINFORCEMENTS

STRETCHING, STRENGTHENING,
AND CROSS-TRAINING

DISCOVERING THE SPORT OF RUNNING is a lot like falling in love. Both make you feel good about yourself, help you enjoy your body, and make you feel sexy. You run because the sport, like your mate, has become part of you. Life without it would be unimaginable.

Loyalty is an important component of both love and running, with one key difference: Sampling other forms of exercise makes your running stronger (as opposed to what "sampling" other men could do to your marriage). Cross-training can give you a solid cardiovascular workout while allowing your joints and muscles a break from the impact of running and the discomforts of pregnancy. "For a person who plans to run for a long time, it would behoove her to mix in some low-impact activities," says Geralyn Coopersmith, C.S.C.S., exercise physiologist and owner of Physique Fitness in Ridgefield, Connecticut. Stretching and strength training should be included among those low-impact activities.

STRETCHING AND STRENGTHENING
FOR PREGNANT RUNNERS

Runners seem to be divided down the middle: those who swear by stretching and those who want to swear *at* it. The same goes for strength training. Regardless of which category you fall into, you should understand that the muscles of your pregnant body lengthen and weaken in some places and shorten and tighten in others. A good stretching and strength-building program can counteract some of these changes and keep you running with few problems.

Stretching Exercises

Not only does stretching make sense for your running by helping you avoid injury, it can ease some of the tension and pressure in your crowded body. Always warm up for 5 to 10 minutes before stretching. Just about any light aerobic activity will do. You can also perform your stretching routine after a run, when your muscles are still warm.

"S" Is for Soreness

You may never have imagined that your body would create a giant "S" once you became pregnant, but it will unless you pay attention. Your heavy, forward-tilting pelvis coaxes your lower back into an arch. Your upper back rounds out a bit. Your shoulders rotate inward and your neck strains as you hold your head up. Down below, your widening pelvis may cause your knees and feet to roll inward. Your knees may hyperextend as though they are pointing out through the backs of your legs. All of this can cause a multitude of aches and pains.

By adjusting your posture, you can offset some of these problems. Unfurl your spinal "S" by tucking in your tailbone and rotating your breastbone up and back a few degrees. Your shoulders will follow. (Don't try to lead with your shoulders or you'll pull yourself out of alignment.) Tuck in your chin slightly. Redistribute weight from the inside of your arches to the middle, and unlock your knees. Maintaining good posture while sitting, standing, walking, and running is one of the simplest ways to ward off pains, strains, and injuries.

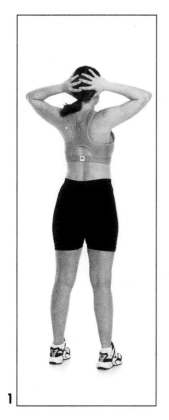

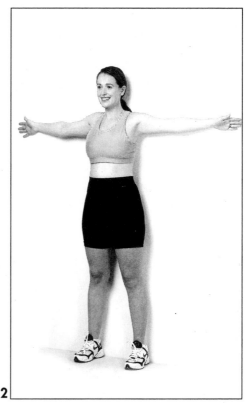

1

2

Chest

To prevent dowager's hump in your upper back, stretch your chest muscles, which shorten and tighten with pregnancy. (1) Stand with your feet shoulder-width apart. Place your hands behind your head with your elbows out. Pull your shoulder blades together and hold for a count of 10. Release and repeat three times.

(2) For an even greater stretch, flatten your back against a wall while holding your arms perpendicular to your body. The palms of your hands should face out. Hold for a count of 10 and release. Repeat three times.

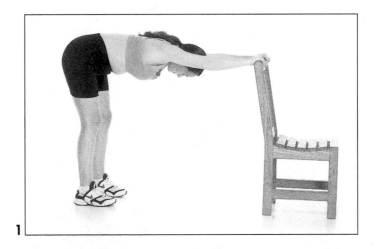

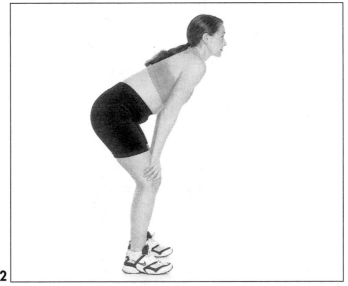

Back

Stretch your upper- and lower-back muscles to offset the tugging from your belly.
(1) To stretch your upper back: With your head tucked between your arms, grab on
to a banister, doorknob, or other stable object that's about waist-high. Bend your
knees slightly and pull away from the object.

(2) To stretch your lower back: Stand with your legs about shoulder-width apart,
bend your knees, and clasp your thighs just above your knees. Check that your knees
are not rolling inward. Keep your back flat so that it is neither hunched nor arched,
and tuck your tailbone under you until you feel a stretch in your lower back. Hold
for 3 to 5 seconds and repeat five times throughout the day.

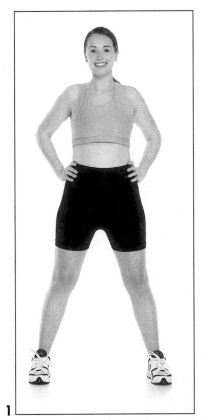

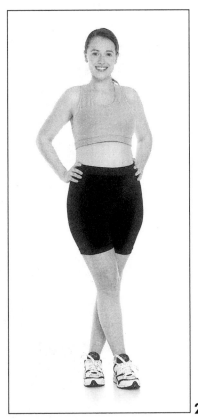

1   2

Outer Thighs and Knees

Instead of a standard stretch, try a grapevine motion. Grapevines gently stretch your abductor muscles on the outsides of your thighs and your iliotibial bands, which run from your hips along the outsides of your thighs to your knees. (1) Place your hands on your hips. Take a big step sideways with your right foot so that your feet are at least 2 feet apart.

(2) Cross behind it with your left foot. Then continue by taking another big step sideways with your right foot and crossing in front of it with your left. After 5 to 10 steps (or when you run out of room), switch directions. Repeat 10 times.

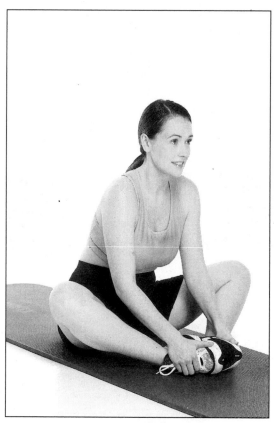

Butterfly

Sit on the floor and maintain good posture by tucking your tailbone under and keeping your lower back from slouching. Bend your knees and place the soles of your feet together, allowing your knees to open to the sides. Hold your feet with your hands. Maintain the position for 20 seconds and repeat once. Increase the stretch by leaning forward from the hips with your back straight. Never force a stretch, especially around the pelvic area.

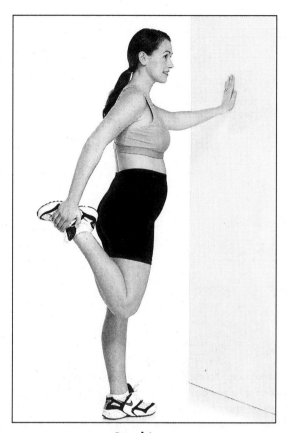

Quadriceps

Your thigh muscles will tighten under the weight of your belly. Here's a familiar exercise to loosen them up. Support yourself by holding on to a wall or another stationary object. Pull your left heel to your buttocks, then move it forward slightly until you feel the stretch in the front of your thigh. Keep your right leg straight without locking your knee. Tuck your tailbone under slightly so that your pelvis is in a neutral position, and try not to arch your back. Hold for a count of 10. Switch legs and repeat three times on each side.

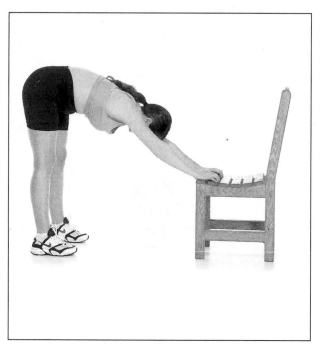

Hamstrings

Running shortens and tightens your hamstrings whether you're pregnant or not. This yoga exercise is known as the modified downward facing dog. Stand with your feet shoulder-width apart about 2 feet from a stationary object, such as a bench. Bend forward at your hips and rest your hands on the bench. Keep your butt in the air and your back straight—don't tuck your tailbone under or hunch your shoulders—and feel the stretch in the backs of your thighs. Bend your knees slightly if you need to, but the straighter your legs, the better the stretch. Check that your feet don't roll inward. Hold the stretch for 10 seconds. Repeat three times.

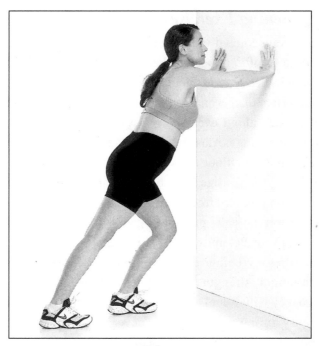

Calves

As your pregnancy progresses, the shift in your gait will tighten your calf muscles. Stand about 2 feet from a wall, extend one leg behind you, and place your weight on that leg so that your foot rests flat on the floor. Allow your forward leg to bend. Lean with your hands against the wall, arms slightly bent. You will feel the calf of your back leg stretching. Hold for a count of 10. Switch legs and repeat three times on each side. To increase the stretch, shift your pelvis slightly forward.

Strengthening Exercises

You've always known that strength training boosts your running power and staves off injury. Now that you're pregnant, a different combination of muscles supports your body, and reinforcing those muscles is more important than ever. The pelvic floor muscles, for example, are essential for just about everything, says Joy Backstrum, a physical therapist in Anchorage, Alaska. "Before you even raise your arm over your head, your pelvic floor and your abdominal and lumbar stabilizers are contracting to stabilize your base of support," she says. During pregnancy, with pressure from the additional weight of the baby, these muscles—specifically the pubococcygeal (PC) muscles—play an important role. (Your PC muscles are the ones you use to stop and start your urine flow.) Whether or not you plan to undertake a strength-training program, strengthen your pelvic floor muscles throughout your pregnancy with Kegel exercises to help maintain bladder control, reduce injury during delivery, and recover more quickly postpartum. (For detailed Kegel exercises, see chapter 10.)

The following simple exercises will work the other key areas of your body. Make sure you warm up with light aerobic activity for 5 to 10 minutes—or complete your run—before you strength-train.

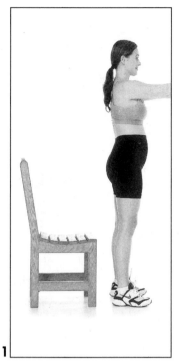
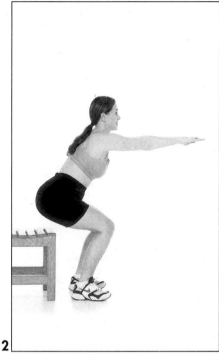

Functional Squats

These modified squats strengthen the deep muscles around the hips. They'll help you later in pregnancy with basic functions like getting in and out of chairs. Strong hip muscles help minimize the third-trimester shuffle. As a runner, you'll also enjoy the power these exercises can build in your quads, hamstrings, and glutes. (1) Stand with your back to a chair or sturdy footstool with your feet shoulder-width apart or slightly wider. Make sure that your toes point forward and your knees do not roll inward. Hold your arms out in front of you for balance.

(2) Squat deeply, as though you are about to sit down, but stop an inch or two above the chair—your thighs will be slightly above parallel to the floor. Lean your torso over your thighs at about a 90-degree angle. Hold for 2 seconds and return to the standing position. Work up to 15 to 20 squats a day. Feel free to take away the chair after you master the exercise.

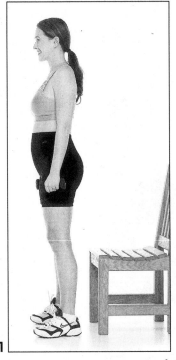
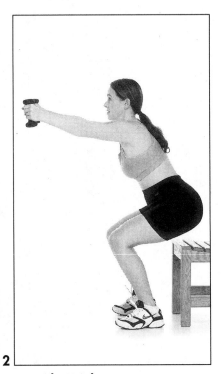

1 2

Functional Squats with Weights

(1) For a more challenging squat variation, hold a dumbbell in each hand or strap on wrist weights. (Start with 1- to 2-pound weights and increase the weight gradually as you gain strength. Stop the exercise if you feel any muscle strain.)

(2) Squat deeply as described on page 45. Bring your arms up to shoulder level and out in front of you.

For another variation, instead of holding your arms in front of you, bring them up diagonally (about halfway between out to your sides and in front) to ear level. Face your thumbs toward the ceiling. Hold for 2 seconds and slowly bring your arms down as you return to the standing position. Work up to 15 to 20 a day.

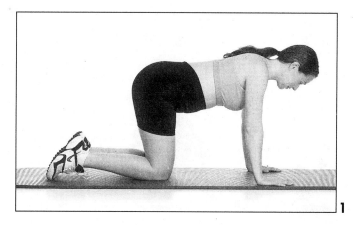

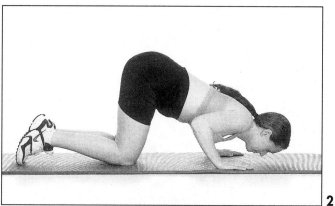

Yoga Pushup

This is the easiest version. (1) Get on your hands and knees with your thighs perpendicular to the floor. Find a neutral position for your pelvis and keep your back straight. Tuck in your chin slightly.

(2) Bend your arms and let your forehead come within an inch or two of the floor. Hold the position for 2 seconds and come up. Repeat 10 times and work up to three sets of 20.

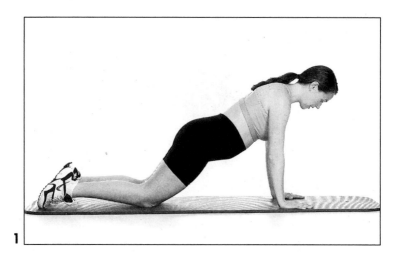

1

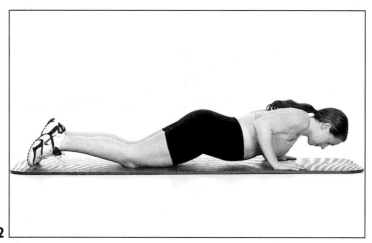

2

"Girl" Pushup

This pushup employs more of your body weight. (1) Get on your hands and knees but "walk" forward with your hands until your thighs are about 45 degrees from the floor. Rest your shins on the floor, keep your pelvis in a neutral position with your back straight, and tuck in your chin.

(2) Bend your arms and lower your forehead to within 2 to 3 inches of the floor (or as far as you can go without your belly touching). Hold for 2 seconds and push back up again. Repeat 10 times and work up to three sets of 20.

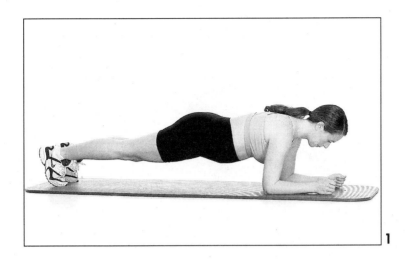

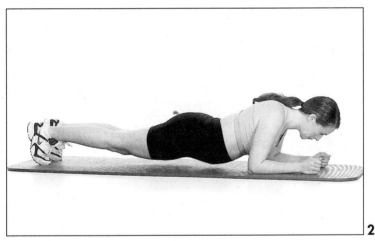

The Plank

Still not challenged? Try this modification. (1) Get into the standard pushup position, but rest your forearms flat on the floor, shoulder-width apart. Keep your back straight. Your face will be 4 to 5 inches from the floor.

(2) Dip your arms until your face comes within 2 inches of the floor. Return to the starting position. Try one and rest. Work up to 10 or more in a day. Most pregnant women do not perform this exercise past the second trimester.

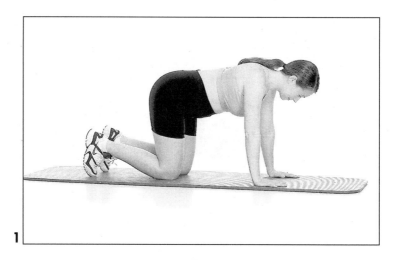

1

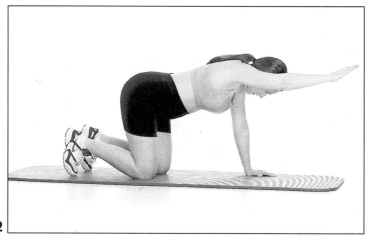

2

Quadruped

The back extensor muscles that run along your spine help support your heavy load up front. (1) Rest on your hands and knees with your head and neck in line with your back. Inhale. As you exhale, imagine drawing your belly button to your spine.

(2) At the same time, reach forward with your right arm so that it forms a straight line with your back, and hold for a count of two. Bring your arm back down and repeat on the other side. Concentrate on keeping your back straight, not arched, as gravity tugs at your belly. When you can complete five repetitions on each side with ease, you're ready to move on to your legs.

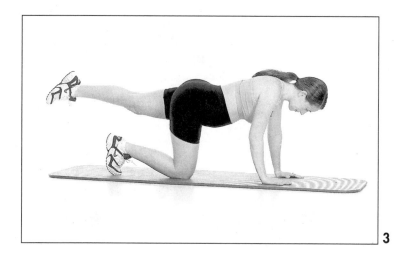

3

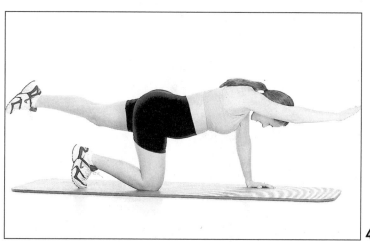

4

(3) Point one leg straight behind you so that it is in line with your back. Hold it still for a count of two and release. Repeat on each side five times.

(4) When you become comfortable with the arm and leg portions of this exercise and can perform them without your muscles shaking, combine them to lift one arm along with the opposite leg. Hold for a count of two, and repeat the exercise 10 times on each side. Work up to two sets of 25 repetitions.

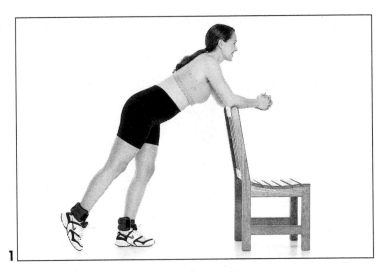

1

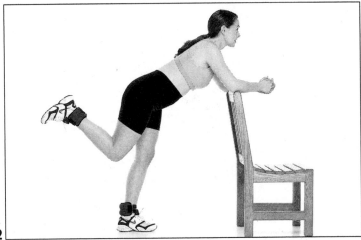

2

Leg Curls

When the hip extensor muscles (the gluteus maximus and the hamstrings) are weak, your back takes up the slack and you can wind up with backaches. (1) Strap on a pair of 2½-pound or 5-pound ankle weights. Stand 2 to 3 feet away from the back of a chair or other sturdy piece of furniture. Leaning forward from your hips, rest your forearms on top of the object. Contract your abdominal muscles and buttocks, and keep your back straight. Extend your right foot behind you and rest your toes on the floor.

(2) Bend your right knee, pulling your foot toward your buttocks slowly. Then release. (Count to two as you raise your leg and to two as you lower it.) Do three sets of 10 repetitions on each side. If you do not have ankle weights or you find the exercise too challenging, you can perform it without the weights.

CROSS-TRAINING FOR PREGNANT RUNNERS

Whether you're accomplished in a number of sports or new to anything but running, remember to follow common sense when it comes to cross-training: If you feel your heavy belly crowding your bladder, don't jump and kick through an aerobics class. If getting to the pool after work means fighting nail-biting traffic, find a new pool or another sport.

And if you're new to a sport don't try to perform at the same level you run—being in good running condition in no way guarantees that you can cycle or cross-country ski to your heart's content. Your body is geared up for the exercise you do the most. "It's called *specificity of training*," says Coopersmith. So start slowly with cross-training and build, just as you did when you first started running. Pay attention to how your body feels, and stop or slow down if you become uncomfortable.

Swimming

Water offers powerful resistance for a challenging whole-body workout. Best of all, it makes you feel light even when you're not. "I always encourage people to swim if they know how," says Mcaire Trapp, a Winnetka, Illinois, triathlete and mother of three. "It's so gentle on your body, and you can do it through your whole pregnancy."

Use any stroke that makes you comfortable and gives you a good workout. The breaststroke in particular can build the deep musculature in your hips and help prevent injury. Freestyle works your upper body, which is good for your posture.

If you feel inefficient in the water, find a coach or experienced swimmer to evaluate your style and suggest improvements. Kicking correctly is especially important. Kicks that are too deep or too wide can cause pelvic pain, a problem that could plague you throughout your pregnancy and beyond. Stop and change strokes the moment you sense pain. And expect to slow down. "As my pregnancy progressed, I went into slower and slower lanes and soon I was in the very slowest lane," says Wendy Gellert, an Anchorage, Alaska, runner and mother of two. "But that was okay. I was still getting a workout, and it was a nice alternative."

Water Wisdom

Pregnant women swear by water sports. Slipping into a pool instantly lightens the load of a baby-packed belly, the hydrostatic pressure can ease swelling in your feet and ankles, and the water tends to keep your body cooler. But before you suit up, keep these things in mind.

- Enter a pool gently by using the ladder or sliding off the edge. Never jump (in case water is forced into your vagina) or dive, which can cause impact to the baby.

- If you are exercising strenuously, make sure the water is below 86°F. Even if it is, you still may sweat during a hard workout.

- If you track your heart rate, understand that water can cause it to drop by up to 17 beats per minute, even when you're working very hard.

- Pay attention to your posture when doing water aerobics or deep-water running: Don't allow your shoulders to creep toward your ears; hold them back slightly and keep your chest high while tucking your tailbone underneath you. "Reevaluate your form every couple of minutes," says Christine Cornell, a prenatal water fitness instructor at Central Dupage Hospital in Winfield, Illinois.

During the third trimester, use caution when doing the breaststroke or using a kickboard, since both cause you to arch—and possibly to strain—your back. The horizontal position of swimming also may aggravate heartburn.

Water Aerobics

Like swimming, water aerobics provides a total-body workout. Classes abound—you can find them at almost any public or health-club pool. As with land-based aerobics, there are many different types: shallow-end, deep-end, choreographed, nonchoreographed, and prenatal, as well as classes that include actual swimming or water running. Some classes concentrate on strength building as opposed to a cardiovascular workout.

Not only does the water make your pregnant body feel good, but you can exercise in positions that would be ridiculous on land. The water resistance allows you to work as hard or as easily as you wish. Most pregnant exercisers use a buoyant device such as a vest, which can be opened to accommodate a growing belly; an adjustable flotation belt; or a flotation noodle—a flexible polyethylene foam tube that makes it easy to rotate and stay put. Whichever device you use, it should keep you from tipping forward or backward and from treading to stay afloat. If the device rides up and irritates your armpits, readjust it until it feels comfortable, even if it means getting out of the water. All of these things will affect your posture and the quality of your workout. Before attending a class, contact the instructor or an employee at the pool to find out if the facility provides flotation devices. Many do.

Strength-training classes sometimes incorporate water dumbbells. Dumbbells are terrific for upper-body workouts but can aggravate carpal tunnel syndrome, a fairly common problem for pregnant women. Keep a soft enough grasp on the equipment so that you can wiggle your fingers, or grip with your thumb and forefinger only.

Deep-Water Running

Deep-water running works the same muscles as land-based running, but with no impact and no belly bounce. That's good for joints and ligaments, not to mention your comfort level. You need two things for this type of cross-training: a pool deep enough so that your feet won't touch bottom and a buoyant device (like the ones mentioned above) to keep you vertical and submerged to just under your shoulders. Many pregnant women prefer belts, which are designed for water running and, in many cases, can be adjusted to accommodate a 48-inch waist. Some belts can be tethered to the side of the pool to enhance the workout as you "run away" from shore. Be sure your belt fits comfortably.

When you run in the water, try to mimic your regular stride. Move your arms at the shoulder joint, and lift each knee to just below your waist. Fighting boredom may be your biggest challenge, so find a buddy or join a class. If you find the workouts too difficult at first, start by walking in the shallow end and graduate to running.

Walking

Let's face it—most of us don't think of walking as *real* exercise. It's what we use to warm up or cool down. Here are four simple modifications that transform it from wimpy to worthwhile.

1. Just being pregnant gives you an added cardiovascular benefit. You're circulating higher blood volume and your heart pushes more blood through the vessels with each beat. Simple walking becomes more strenuous, especially later in pregnancy when you're front-loaded with an additional 15 pounds.

2. If you walk on a treadmill, you can design a very strenuous workout. Judy Gower, a triathlon coach in Anchorage, Alaska, suggests setting the treadmill at a 12 percent grade and walking at a fast clip. "It's really good exercise and there's no pounding," she says.

3. Go for a hike. The hillier the trail, the better the workout.

4. Walk quickly, especially if you don't have access to hills. You don't have to speedwalk; just increase the pace until you can feel yourself breathing harder. Concentrate on picking up your feet a little higher off the ground—you won't trip and you'll give your legs a better workout.

Group Exercise Classes

The array of options is dizzying. In general, classes fall into three categories.

High-impact aerobics: Some of the trendier classes like kickboxing and boot camps are considered high-impact, along with other classes that require hopping or jumping movements. High-impact aerobic exercisers keep pace with fast music that reaches 150 beats per minute or higher.

If you've already been doing high-impact aerobics, you probably can continue well into your pregnancy, barring any problems. But classes that require high kicks and fast side-to-side movements may cause problems later on. Your big belly will limit the range of your

Four Tips for Doing Aerobics While Pregnant

Aerobic-exercise classes are an ideal cross-training option during pregnancy. The benefits aren't just for you—your baby may enjoy the rocking motion and the sound of the music. Here's how to get the most from your workout.

1. Avoid quick directional changes and side-to-side moves as well as spinning motions unless you've been doing aerobics for a long time and are confident in your balance. Ask the instructor to help you substitute simpler moves if necessary.

2. Fitness rooms can get hot. If you feel you are overheating, take a break and leave the room.

3. Keep a water bottle within reach.

4. You don't have to show up in tight-fitting clothes. Most people wear shorts and T-shirts.

high kicks, and your fleeting sense of balance can send you for a tumble when you stride sideways.

If you want to try high-impact aerobics and it's early in your pregnancy, give it a whirl. But proceed with caution, and if you begin to feel exhausted or sore, take a rest.

Low-impact aerobics: Low-impact aerobics means that at least one foot stays grounded, and the music beat is slower, usually around 140 beats per minute. Again, beware of lateral movements.

Step aerobics is a popular low-impact form of aerobics. Participants use a platform that ranges in height from 4 to 8 inches. Some women discard the step altogether in late pregnancy and perform the exercises on the floor to avoid tripping (easy to do when your belly blocks your view).

Prenatal exercise: Prenatal exercise classes place a higher priority on pregnancy issues than on cardiovascular fitness. Instructors concentrate on stretching, body alignment, and exercises that strengthen pelvic muscles. Classes vary greatly, depending upon the instructor and the fitness level of people in the class.

Runners sometimes dismiss prenatal exercise classes when, in fact, these classes offer complementary benefits to regular training. If you decide to sign up, call the instructor ahead of time to find out her philosophy and what you can expect from the class. And don't minimize the importance of meeting other pregnant women—you may even find a running buddy.

Cycling

No other sport can give your body a break from the pounding of running, boost your VO_2 max, and build superb strength in your quadriceps and glutes like cycling can. It's a low-impact sport—unless you crash. That's why most pregnant athletes opt for stationary bikes after their balance begins to shift, usually around the fourth or fifth month.

Running legs are not the same as cycling legs. It takes time to achieve cycling fitness, and your muscles will begin to tire much earlier in a cycling workout than in a running workout. That's because even though you use some of the same muscles, you use them differently. Start with slower and easier rotations until you build strength and the workouts become less taxing. When you get into better shape, remember that cycling has a 4-to-1 ratio to running. In other words, 4 miles of cycling equals 1 mile of running.

As your belly expands, the biomechanics of your cycling will change, and you'll have to

Sports to Avoid While Pregnant:

- Downhill skiing
- Water skiing
- Horseback riding
- Scuba diving
- Skydiving and hang gliding
- Contact sports
- Any exercise performed at more than 10,000 feet and in temperatures over 85°F

pedal around your belly, with knees and hips rotating outward. Some women switch to recumbent stationary bikes late in pregnancy because sitting upright can put pressure on the bladder, bowel, lungs, and stomach.

Group cycling fitness classes can help chase away the boredom of stationary cycling and provide a worthwhile workout. If you attend such a class, don't try to keep up with your nonpregnant neighbors. Limit out-of-the-saddle drills, since standing and peddling can put extra pressure on your knees. Check out the room ahead of time to make sure it has adequate ventilation and plenty of fans: Stationary cycling creates a lot of sweat and no breeze, and a group cycling room can quickly feel like a sauna.

Clothing note: Maternity workout clothing catalogs and Web sites carry high-quality bike shorts (see the Resource Guide).

Cross-Country Skiing

Cross-country skiing provides a low-impact, whole-body workout with special emphasis on increasing muscle strength and flexibility in the hip area. Muscles around the hips play a vital role in holding up your bulging abdomen, and they become less flexible during pregnancy. The constant flexing and extending of the legs in cross-country skiing will help improve your range of motion.

As with running, cross-country skiing brings you outside and gives you a chance to enjoy the view. In places where snow is plentiful, cross-country skiing is sometimes a more logical choice for exercise, and many of the women interviewed for this book switched over entirely during the winter. "During my first pregnancy, I quit running," says Gellert. "The snow was great, and it was a really good winter for skiing. I could have run more, but I didn't need to."

Pregnant athletes usually stick to classical-style cross-country skiing, where the skis run parallel to each other. The other style is called *skate skiing*, and it uses the same side-to-side motion that downhill skiers use when traveling between chairlifts. Except for advanced skate skiers, most women should avoid this type of skiing during pregnancy because it requires greater balance and stamina.

If you're new to cross-country skiing, rent the skis, poles, and boots the first time out. Take a class. Be careful around hills and trees; they can be a dangerous combination for new skiers, especially those with less-than-perfect balance. "Watch your terrain," Coopersmith says. "You don't want to risk a fall. If you do fall, try to land on your side or your buttocks."

Wear layered clothing made from synthetic fabrics that draw sweat away from your skin, as well as a hat and gloves, and stay hydrated. Always ski with a partner or group, unless you're skiing somewhere you can summon help quickly.

Clothing note: Pregnant cross-country skiers complain of clothes that ride up and result in cold bellies. A maternity unitard (or a regular one that you stretch out) can help, especially if it's underneath a pair of warm fleece pants that envelop your belly. Wear a jacket or long shirt over the pants to hide the W. C. Fields look.

Exercise Machines

If you belong to a gym, these three machines are among the safest and most effective for your pregnant body.

Stairclimbers: Stairclimbing is a low-impact, weight-bearing form of exercise. It helps build power in the quadriceps muscles, an added benefit to your running. Plan a workout equal in duration to your regular run, but begin with the machine on a low setting (shallow steps instead of deep ones). Most stairclimbers allow you to adjust the intensity in the middle of your session, so readjust it if you feel the need. Work toward deeper steps as you become accustomed to the equipment.

Watch your posture while on the stairclimber. Use the handrails and stand upright. If you lean forward, you risk injuring your back during pregnancy. Correct posture will also help bolster your buttocks and back muscles.

Elliptical trainers: Elliptical trainers provide a no-impact workout with loads of variety: forward and backward rotations, different resistance levels, and high and low grades. Some machines also include moving poles that allow you to work your upper body.

During your second and third trimesters, you will need to pay attention to your posture on the elliptical trainer, as back strain is a very real threat, especially if you're using the upper-body workout features.

Cross-country ski machines: No snow in your part of the country? You can get some of the same benefits by using indoor equipment. If you belong to a gym or health club in which you can use a ski machine, have one of the employees show you how to adjust it for your size and fitness level. Ski machines can take a few tries before you find the right rhythm, but they are worth the effort. *User tip:* Most machines have a waist pad to rest against; if you're shifting most of your weight to the pad, you're likely pressing too hard.

Yoga

Yoga, an ancient Hindu system of precise posture and breathing, can reduce stress, relieve pain, and improve your stamina and sense of well-being. It can also help you prevent injury by increasing your flexibility. The poses and postures will challenge your strength, while going easy on your joints. You can safely perform most of the poses during pregnancy.

You can find several books and videos on yoga for pregnancy or yoga for running. A number of women interviewed for this book took regular yoga classes and continued throughout their pregnancies, with a few modifications. Finding a class is as easy as scanning the yellow pages.

Pilates

Developed more than 70 years ago by German gymnast, boxer, and circus performer Joseph Pilates, this form of exercise develops strength, flexibility, and balance. It's a good enhancement to your regular aerobic workout.

Pilates exercises both stretch and strengthen the rectus abdominis—a muscle group that will help support your baby. That means if you learn to do the exercises correctly you may ward off back pain and other injuries common to pregnant athletes. Pilates exercises increase blood flow to your abdominal area, and presumably your uterus, which benefits the baby by bringing him more oxygen.

Some other benefits of Pilates:

- Greater awareness of your body, leading to better balance and coordination during pregnancy

- Broader range of motion as your muscles stretch and lengthen

- Improved posture, which will offset the tugging on your spine by the baby

You can learn the exercises on your own through books or videos (at least one book and one video have been produced specifically on Pilates during pregnancy). Or visit your local Pilates studio and ask about classes.

NUTRITION

EATING FOR TWO ON THE RUN

NEXT TIME YOU SIT DOWN AT THE DINNER TABLE, imagine yourself as a car pulling into a filling station. As you eat, remember that your "fuel tank" supplies both your running and your pregnancy, not to mention your day-to-day living. That makes it necessary to consume high-grade foods in amounts that leave you satisfied. Carefully plan your meals and snacks and commit yourself to eating healthfully.

"A good pregnancy diet and a good runner's diet intersect 100 percent," says Nancy Clark, R.D., author of *Nancy Clark's Sports Nutrition Guidebook* and a nutrition counselor at SportsMedicine Associates in Brookline, Massachusetts. "As a runner and as a pregnant woman, you want to fuel your body optimally," she says. That means designing a food plan based on fruits and vegetables, whole grains, proteins, and calcium-rich foods.

Nutritional needs will vary slightly throughout pregnancy. "The first trimester, when most of the cell division is going on, is when a pregnant woman needs vitamins and micronutrients the most, especially folic acid and zinc," says Robert E. Keith, R.D., Ph.D., professor of nutrition and food science at Auburn University in Alabama. To be on the safe side, take a prenatal multivitamin supplement even if you eat a nutrient-rich diet and hate the thought of popping a tablet. A prenatal vitamin will not only cover your baby's nutritional needs but also provide a superior source of folic acid. The body absorbs folic acid from supplements more readily than it absorbs the folate found naturally in food. Your doctor can prescribe a prenatal supplement or may recommend an over-the-counter variety.

In terms of caloric needs, experts advise pregnant women to consume about 2,300 calories a day. And here's the fun part: As a pregnant *runner*, you can pile another 100 calories per mile onto your plate! You already should be eating a combination of 55 to 60 percent of calories from carbohydrates, 25 to 30 percent from fat, and 10 to 15 percent from protein.

Foods That Do Double Duty

A few highly nutritious foods will furnish your growing baby and your runner's body.

	BEANS	LENTILS	ORANGES	BANANAS	SWEET POTATOES	WHITE POTATOES	WHOLE-GRAIN BREAD	YOGURT	MILK
Protein	X	X						X	X
Carbohydrates	X	X	X	X	X	X	X	X	X
Water			X						X
Fiber	X	X		X	X	X	X		
Vitamin A					X				
Folic acid	X	X	X						
Vitamin C			X		X	X			
Calcium								X	X
Iron	X								
Potassium	X			X	X	X			

Because you're balancing the needs of your pregnancy and your sport, pay extra attention to protein and carbohydrates. "Protein is a significant component of a growing baby," says Dr. Keith. "If a pregnant woman doesn't eat protein, her body will be broken down to supply the needs of the fetus." If you're a distance runner, you probably already eat complex carbohydrates to keep your glycogen stores high. That's good for your pregnancy because your body converts carbohydrates into glucose, and your baby uses glucose as his main energy source.

Staying Hydrated

Both pregnancy and running tax your body's hydration levels. Drink enough liquid so that your urine runs clear, the volume is high, and you have to go every 2 to 4 hours. Some of your fluid intake can be water, and some can be milk or fruit juice. "Fruit juices contain carbohydrates and lots of vitamins and minerals," says Dr. Keith. "By drinking them, you can also meet some of your caloric needs."

Unfortunately, if you're prone to morning sickness, you may trigger nausea every time you drink fluids. Try drinking just a few sips at a time and drinking after small snacks or meals. Stay away from beverages that seem unappealing.

Many runners rely on nonnutritive substances to sustain them. Caffeine is a popular performance enhancer but doctors don't recommend it during pregnancy, as it can increase the risk of miscarriage. Some sports gels contain caffeine, so read the label before you take one.

SO WHAT SHOULD YOU EAT?

Following are a week's worth of nutritionist-approved, healthy, realistic meals to sustain your baby, your health, and your running. Each day's meals total between 2,300 and 2,500 calories, so you may need to adjust serving sizes to meet your specific energy needs.

This meal plan is not a diet—it is simply a guideline for healthy eating during pregnancy. Feel free to add, eliminate, or substitute foods based on your appetite and preferences. For instance, if you can't stand fat-free milk, try 1%; if you're lactose intolerant, exchange the dairy selections for soy; if you're not a dessert person, eat an extra portion of your main meal. Don't forget your prenatal vitamin supplements. And, of course, check with your obstetrician before following these or any other nutritional guidelines.

Beginning on page 72 I've included a shopping list. If you photocopy it and tuck it into your tote bag, you'll set grocery-shopping speed records—and have that much more time to hit the trail!

AT-A-GLANCE MEAL SUGGESTIONS FOR PREGNANT RUNNERS

Day 1

Breakfast
1 cup unsweetened, high-fiber breakfast cereal, such as Multi-Bran Chex, with ½ cup fat-free milk, 1 banana, ¼ cup berries, and 1 teaspoon honey
Water, decaf iced or hot tea, or other low-calorie beverage

Snack
2 ounces (1-inch cube) Cheddar cheese
1 apple

Lunch
1 cup beef, turkey, or vegetarian chili with ¼ cup parsley (mix the parsley into heated chili for added vitamin C, amino acids, potassium, and folate)
1 small baked potato, plain
1 cup fat-free milk

Snack
2 ounces small pretzel sticks (about 95 sticks)
2 tablespoons hummus
1 cup orange juice

Dinner

Salad made with 1 cup mixed salad greens; 1 carrot, thinly sliced; 2 tablespoons salad dressing; and 3 ounces diced chicken (white meat is fine, but dark meat, such as from the thigh, has more iron and zinc)
2 slices whole grain toast with 1 tablespoon margarine
Water, decaf iced or hot tea, or other low-calorie beverage

Dessert

1 cup rice pudding

TOTAL CALORIES: 2,400

Day 2

Breakfast

½ cup cottage cheese
½ cup berries or kiwifruit
1 whole grain bagel with 2 tablespoons cream cheese
1 cup cranberry juice

Snack

1 baked sweet potato, plain
10 Triscuit crackers
Water, decaf iced or hot tea, or other low-calorie beverage

Lunch

1 slice pizza with vegetable toppings, such as green bell peppers, mushrooms, onions, et cetera
1 cup mixed greens with dressing made of 2 teaspoons balsamic or red wine vinegar and 1 tablespoon olive oil
1 small whole wheat dinner roll
1 cup fat-free milk

Snack

2 oatmeal cookies
1 cup fat-free milk

Dinner

3 ounces grilled or baked fish or other seafood (avoid swordfish, shark, and marlin, and limit your intake of fresh tuna to one serving a week—these fish may contain harmful mercury levels; check with your doctor for more details)
1 cup cooked long-grain or brown rice
1 cup grilled or steamed asparagus

Salad made with 2 cups romaine lettuce, 20 whole wheat croutons, and
   2 tablespoons dressing
Water, decaf iced or hot tea, or other low-calorie beverage

Dessert
¾ cup vanilla frozen yogurt
¼ cup granola

TOTAL CALORIES: 2,560

Day 3

Breakfast
2 slices whole grain toast with 2 tablespoons peanut butter
1 kiwifruit
1 cup fat-free milk

Snack
1 cup plain yogurt with 1 teaspoon jam and ¼ cup berries, chopped banana, or other favorite fruit
1 cup apple juice

Lunch
2 open-faced broiled sandwiches, each made with 1 slice whole grain
   bread, ½ ounce cheese, and 1 thick tomato slice
1 cup grapes
Water, decaf iced or hot tea, or other low-calorie beverage

Snack
1 carrot
1 tablespoon ranch, dill, or other flavor dip
6 small sesame sticks
1 cup cranberry juice

Dinner
4 ounces steak
1 grilled red bell pepper, sliced
1 cup steamed broccoli
1 or 2 boiled red potatoes with 1 teaspoon margarine
1 cup fat-free milk

Dessert
1 slice apple pie

TOTAL CALORIES: 2,445

Day 4

Breakfast
1 hard-boiled egg
1 cup fresh fruit, such as strawberries, blueberries, banana, or kiwifruit
1 slice toast with 1 teaspoon jam
1 cup fat-free milk

Snack
½ cup Multi-Bran Chex cereal mixed with ¼ cup almonds, cashews, peanuts, walnuts, or other nuts
1 cup orange juice

Lunch
Sandwich made with 2 slices whole grain bread, 2 thick or 3 thin slices turkey, 2 romaine lettuce leaves, and 2 teaspoons mustard or 1 tablespoon mayonnaise
1 cup low-fat (baked) potato or corn chips
1 carrot
Water, decaf iced or hot tea, or other low-calorie beverage

Snack
Chocolate milk made with 1 cup fat-free milk and 1 teaspoon chocolate powder

Dinner
1 cup cooked spaghetti
½ cup spaghetti sauce
3 or 4 small meatballs
Salad made with 1 cup fresh spinach, 2 tablespoons grated Parmesan cheese, and 2 tablespoons salad dressing
Water, decaf iced or hot tea, or other low-calorie beverage

Dessert
1 piece fruit crisp, such as peach, berry, or apple

TOTAL CALORIES: 2,345

Day 5

Breakfast
1 bran muffin
1 cup plain yogurt with 1 chopped banana or ½ cup berries
Water, decaf iced or hot tea, or other low-calorie beverage

Snack

¼ cup raisins or other dried fruit
¼ cup sunflower seeds
Water, decaf iced or hot tea, or other low-calorie beverage

Lunch

1 veggie burger on 1 whole grain bun, with 1 slice American or Cheddar
    cheese and 1 to 2 tablespoons ketchup, mustard, or other condiment
½ cup canned corn
Water, decaf iced or hot tea, or other low-calorie beverage

Snack

1 cup V8 juice
1 whole wheat English muffin
1 tablespoon guacamole

Dinner

1 cup chicken or cheese tortellini with ¼ cup marinated sun-dried toma-
    toes and 2 tablespoons grated Parmesan cheese
1 cup steamed broccoli and cauliflower
1 cup fat-free milk

Dessert

1 slice zucchini bread

TOTAL CALORIES: 2,365

Day 6

Breakfast

¾ cup oatmeal mixed with ⅛ cup fat-free milk (to taste) and 1 tablespoon
    maple syrup
1 peach
1 cup orange juice

Snack

Smoothie made with 1 cup fat-free milk, 1 banana, 1 graham cracker
    (4 rectangles), and ½ teaspoon cinnamon

Lunch

1 cup lentil soup
Sandwich made with 2 slices whole grain bread, 2 thin slices ham, and 2
    teaspoons mustard
1 cup apple juice

Snack
Pizza made with 1 pita, ¼ cup shredded mozzarella cheese, and 2 table-
spoons hummus (spread hummus after melting cheese on pita)
Water, decaf iced or hot tea, or other low-calorie beverage

Dinner
4 to 5 ounce pork chop
½ cup applesauce
1 cup brown rice
1 cup steamed green beans with ¼ cup sliced almonds
1 cup fat-free milk

Dessert
1 cup vanilla frozen yogurt
1 tablespoon hot fudge or hot caramel topping

TOTAL CALORIES: 2,425

Day 7

Breakfast
2 6-inch whole wheat pancakes with 1 teaspoon soft margarine and 1 tablespoon maple syrup
1 cup fat-free milk

Snack
2 large slices cantaloupe or other seasonal fruit

Lunch
Sandwich made with 2 slices whole grain bread, 2 ounces water-packed
white tuna, 1 tablespoon mayonnaise, and ⅛ cup diced celery
1 cup tomato soup
10 saltines
Water, decaf iced or hot tea, or other low-calorie beverage

Snack
1 cranberry or blueberry muffin
1 cup fat-free milk

Dinner
1 burrito made with 1 8-inch tortilla, ½ cup refried beans, ¼ cup shredded
Cheddar cheese, and 1 sliced raw, grilled, or marinated green bell pepper
10 corn chips
2 tablespoons salsa
Water, decaf iced or hot tea, or other low-calorie beverage

Dessert

1 slice angel food cake with ¾ cup berries

TOTAL CALORIES: 2,291

SHOPPING LIST

With this grocery list, you can stock your fridge and cupboards for at least a week. Many of the items are staples that you probably already have. Freeze breads and fresh meats and fish, then thaw them on the day you plan to eat them.

Breads/Grains

Bagels, whole grain
Bread, whole grain
Breakfast cereal, unsweetened, such as Multi-Bran Chex, Fruit & Fibre, Grape-Nuts
Croutons, whole wheat
Dinner rolls, whole wheat
English muffins, whole wheat
Granola
Hamburger buns, whole grain
Muffins, bran, plus either blueberry or cranberry
Oatmeal
Pancake mix, whole wheat
Pitas
Pizza, frozen, with vegetable toppings
Rice, long-grain and brown
Tortillas, 8-inch
Zucchini bread or bread mix

Snacks

Almonds, sliced
Chips, potato or corn, baked
Graham crackers
Nuts, whole, such as almonds, peanuts, cashews, walnuts
Pretzel sticks, small
Saltines
Sesame sticks, small
Sunflower seeds
Triscuits

Fruits

Apples
Bananas
Berries, such as blueberries, raspberries, or strawberries
Cantaloupe
Kiwifruit
Peaches
Raisins

Vegetables

Beans, refried, canned
Bell peppers, green and red
Broccoli
Carrots
Cauliflower
Celery
Corn, canned or frozen
Green beans, fresh or frozen
Mixed salad greens
Parsley
Potatoes, red, baking, and sweet
Romaine lettuce
Spinach
Tomatoes, fresh, plus marinated and sun-dried

Meats

Chicken
Fish or other seafood (3 ounces when cooked)
Meatballs, frozen
Pork chops (4 ounces when cooked)
Steak (4 ounces when cooked)
Tuna, canned
Turkey, sliced
Veggie burgers, frozen

Pasta and Soup

Chili, canned: beef, turkey, or vegetarian
Lentil soup, canned
Spaghetti
Tomato soup, canned
Tortellini, chicken or cheese

Condiments and Spreads

Applesauce
Balsamic vinegar
Chocolate-milk powder mix
Cinnamon
Guacamole
Honey
Hot fudge or caramel sauce
Hummus
Jam
Ketchup
Maple syrup
Margarine
Mayonnaise
Mustard
Olive oil
Salad dressing
Salsa
Spaghetti sauce

Desserts

Angel food cake mix
Apple pie, fresh or frozen
Fruit crisp
Oatmeal cookies
Rice pudding
Vanilla frozen yogurt

Beverages

Apple juice
Cranberry juice
Decaffeinated tea bags or unsweetened iced tea mix
Orange juice
V8 juice

Dairy Products

Cheddar or other cheese
Cottage cheese
Cream cheese
Eggs
Milk, fat-free
Mozzarella cheese, shredded
Parmesan cheese, grated
Yogurt, plain, unsweetened

PART 2:
THE FIRST TRIMESTER

CHAPTER 5

THE FIRST MONTH

STOMACH DOING FLIP-FLOPS? IT MUST BE LOVE (OR PREGNANCY)

THE FUNNIEST TELEVISION SHOW I've ever seen was actually a drama in which a male character and a female character were twisted together in a steamy sex scene. When they finished, the woman whispered in his ear with utter certainty, "We just made a baby."

What a hoot! As though the female body sends some immediate, mysterious signal that sperm and egg have met and are making their way to safe lodging in the uterus—and if you're womanly enough, you'll just sense it.

> **PREGNANCY**
> **STEP**BY**STEP**
>
> Month 1: At 4 weeks your 6-miler feels like it always does, but as your own heart and lungs work in concert to help you run, the tiny embryo in your womb is developing primitive lung buds and a tube that will become his heart.

In reality, it's nothing like that when you're trying to conceive. Instead, after each steamy encounter with your husband, you think, "I wonder if that one took." Then you have to wait and see if your period is late. And if it's delayed by even just a day, you start thinking, "Maybe, maybe . . .". You interpret any hint of nausea or breast tenderness as a good sign. Chances are that the cycle will repeat itself a few more times before you feel any true pregnancy symptoms. By then you've made several expensive trips to the drugstore and your trash can has collected a series of disappointing little white sticks minus the pink stripes. Or, if you're like 15 percent of the population, you've become intimate with an infertility specialist and your baby's conception was far more clinical than steamy.

If your race to get pregnant was full of emotional ups and downs, consider what it's like once conception becomes a reality. Here's what's going on during your first month as a pregnant runner.

FEELINGS AND SENSATIONS

Wonder and Confusion

If this is your first pregnancy, you'll undergo a substantial emotional change in these early weeks—transforming from childless person to mom with kid in storage. The reality of your pregnancy will overtake you suddenly and without warning anytime, anywhere. No matter whether you're thrilled or distressed, you'll probably repeat phrases like *This is unbelievable* or *It doesn't seem real* to yourself many times.

The early physical changes will be subtle, but if you're paying attention, you will see immediate effects on your running. "I'd always been very consistent in my times," says Linda Gill, a San Anselmo, California, runner and mother of four. "All of a sudden they were completely off. That's how I knew I was pregnant."

You're more likely to notice your body's signals if you were focused on the conception process rather than if the pregnancy caught you by surprise. But by the time you move into the second month, the symptoms will leave no doubt in your mind about your condition, especially if you are one of the 50 percent of women who suffer from morning sickness. (The good news: Toward the end of the third month some of your symptoms may taper off and make your running easier.)

Personal Record

Running during pregnancy is a means to an end. You run now so that you can run sooner, better, and faster after your baby is born. Even so, don't charge through these 9 months without paying attention. Keep a journal. Someday you'll want to remember this part of your life and recall the details of your running. Believe it or not, it's fun to go back and review all the aches and pains of pregnancy once you no longer feel them. Track your distance or time on the road, how you feel physically and emotionally, what you see, and what you say to the baby. By month 7, when you're losing steam, reading about your accomplishments will inspire you to keep going. And someday the baby may grow into an athlete who wants to know all about the runs he participated in before birth.

Worry

For many women, worry sets in as soon as they get the great news: "What about the time I _____?" We fill in the blank with some "offense" we would never have committed had we known about the pregnancy—drinking a couple of vodka tonics, running to exhaustion, taking a No-Doz. Stay calm and talk to your doctor. It's unlikely that your baby will suffer from your early-pregnancy mistake if you take good care of yourself from here on.

Exhaustion

During her first pregnancy, my sister Anne fell asleep in the bathroom at work. It was an innocent mistake. She sat on the commode, placed her head on the soft toilet paper roll—which suddenly resembled a pillow—and out went the lights.

This could happen to you. Don't wait for your body to switch off. When you have limited free time, you don't want to spend any of it asleep. But pregnancy is not just a state of being; it's also a state of doing. You have to do the right things to support it. Take a Saturday afternoon nap, go to bed an hour early, close the door to your office at lunch and put your head down on your desk. Or be like Anne and choose a quiet, out-of-the-way stall. Just be sure to slip on a pair of shoes that no one will recognize.

YOUR CONCERNS

Warming Up and Cooling Down Properly

An effective warmup transitions your body from a resting state to an active state and helps ensure that your muscles are warm enough to perform without becoming injured. Start by walking for 2 to 5 minutes followed by jogging for another 2 to 5 minutes until you've eased into your regular pregnancy pace.

Joy Backstrum, a physical therapist in Anchorage, Alaska, suggests incorporating some slow, lateral movements into your warmup. Lateral movements fortify the deep musculature of the hips, which help support your increasingly heavy abdomen. Include five or six grapevines (see page 39 for complete description) or other simple sideways movements in your warmup.

After your run, allow at least 5 minutes of slow jogging or walking to return your body to its resting state gradually. An adequate cooldown keeps blood circulating well (instead of pooling in your legs), which helps you avoid dizziness. Lightly stretch at the end of your cooldown—or perform the stretching routine in chapter 3—to prevent injury.

> ## Bitter Pill
>
> Aches and pains are inevitable for runners. Pregnancy doesn't change that, but it does change the way you can deal with them. Most doctors suggest staying away from aspirin and ibuprofen while you're pregnant. Large amounts can interfere with the baby's heart development and blood-clotting ability and cause jaundice in the baby after birth. If you have relied on these or other anti-inflammatory medications to help decrease swelling after an injury, put them away for now and use the RICE treatment—rest, ice, compression, elevation—for injuries. (For more about RICE, see chapter 7.)

Monitoring Exertion

During the first 3 or 4 weeks of pregnancy, your runs may feel the same as ever. Your body is only beginning its process of radical change, and the baby is an embryo too tiny to give you much trouble. On the other hand, you may start to feel out of breath more easily in the first month as your lungs adapt to the pregnancy.

Another scenario: You go out for your 6-miler at full throttle—or so you think. Your time is off by 3, 4, 5 minutes. Well, get used to it. Pregnancy has a way of forcing us to do the right thing, and slowing down is one of them.

Whether you feel breathless, slow, or normal, stay attuned to your exertion. Use the Borg Rating of Perceived Exertion (RPE) detailed in the sidebar on page 82, and stay within the range of 12 to 14 (slightly to moderately hard).

Should you monitor your heart rate during prenatal exercise? Fifteen or 20 years ago, most doctors would have told you to keep your heart rate under 140 beats per minute based on 1985 guidelines from the American College of Obstetricians and Gynecologists. "That was a number they kicked out a long time ago," says Patty Kulpa, M.D., a sports gynecologist from Gig Harbor, Washington. By 1994, heart rate was considered a less reliable measure of exertion in part because it varies throughout pregnancy. The guidelines were revised and the recommended heart rate eliminated.

Nonetheless, many doctors still advise patients with low-risk pregnancies to keep their heart rates under 140, despite the change in recommendations and the introduction of other measurements, such as the Borg RPE. Many runners quit in frustration when they can't get a sufficient workout under these constraints.

If you already wear a monitor and want to continue using it, go ahead. You may simply enjoy knowing your heart rate, and your pregnancy shouldn't stop you. Just be sure to pay close attention to how your workout feels. Ignore or reprogram your monitor's settings so that you're not tempted to run too hard.

The Borg Rating of Perceived Exertion

Developed by Swedish physiologist Gunnar Borg, the Borg Rating of Perceived Exertion (RPE) is a scale many athletes use to gauge the intensity of their workouts. The scale is effective because it is individualized: You match it to your own assessment of how hard you are working. For example, if you normally run an 8-minute 10-K pace and you slow down to 9-minute miles during pregnancy, you may be working just as hard to maintain that slower pace. The Borg RPE measures your exertion—not your speed, not your heart rate, but what the effort costs you.

The scale starts at 6, which measures no exertion, and goes up to 20, which is as hard as you could possibly exercise. Pregnant runners should not run to the point of exhaustion. Stay within the range of 12 to 14 (slightly to moderately hard) to maintain fitness, recommends L. A. Wolfe, Ph.D., a professor of exercise physiology at the School of Physical Health and Education at Queen's University in Kingston, Ontario.

6	No exertion
7	
8	Extremely light
9	Very light
10	
11	Light
12	
13	Somewhat hard
14	
15	Hard (heavy)
16	
17	Very hard
18	
19	Extremely hard
20	Maximal exertion

As you get bigger (well beyond this first month), the torso band may begin to chafe you. If you wear a bra that holds your monitor in place, you may find that the bra quickly becomes too tight. In either case, try this suggestion from Judy Gower, an Anchorage triathlon coach: "Instead of wearing it at the base of your breast, you can place it in the top of your running bra, about 6 inches down from your neckline and right on top of your breast. You will still get a good reading and it's more comfortable." Gower suggests doubling your running bra or wearing a unitard if the monitor seems loose.

Warm-Weather Running

Ten out of 10 doctors agree: Running in the heat when you're pregnant is unwise. During pregnancy your body can dissipate exercise-generated heat in comfortable temperatures. But when you overheat, your blood rushes to your skin as part of your body's cooling mechanism and is pulled away from the uterus, risking harm to your baby. When the thermometer climbs above 85°F, reschedule your run for a cooler time of day or run in an air-conditioned environment, like an indoor track or at the gym on a treadmill.

If you are well-acclimated and the temperature is hovering near 85°F, bring extra water to pour over your head and hydrate well, since dehydration can increase your body's core temperature. To be sure you stay within a safe limit, you can take your rectal or vaginal temperature right after a run. A reading of 102°F is the upper limit, a temperature you don't want your body to reach on a regular basis.

Cold-Weather Running

With a few minor adjustments, you can continue running through winter. Bundle up as usual with a hat, mittens, and layered clothing. Synthetic clothes that wick away sweat are preferable, but creating the perfect cold-weather maternity running outfit can cost you. Be creative. I wore a pair of maternity running tights, a long-sleeve polypropylene undershirt, an extra-large sweatshirt, and an unzipped outer shell. Other cold-weather runners rave about their unitard, which both supports the belly and keeps it warm under running clothes.

(continued on page 86)

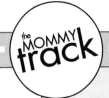

THE GOOD LIFE

Name: Shannon Avery

Birth date: October 1964

Residence: San Juan, Puerto Rico

Occupation: Massage therapist

Children: Two, born 1996 and 1998

NO REASON TO CHANGE

Shannon Avery has a lifestyle most athletic moms envy. She runs 25 to 30 miles a week, cross-trains, lifts weights, does yoga, and meditates. There's one catch: She starts each day at 4:30 (that's A.M.). "Is that crazy or what?" she says.

Her crazy schedule began long before her first pregnancy, and she saw no reason to tone it down for 9 months. "I felt it was better to keep going with the routine I was already used to," she says. "I just wanted to keep my body in the same good state I'd started in." She cut back her mileage to 15 to 20 miles per week through her pregnancy. To combat fatigue, she ate extra protein and snuck in an afternoon nap when she could.

Her training regimen paid off. "My body was beautiful—and not fat like I'd expected it to be," she says.

Her doctor, on the other hand, worried she was jeopardizing her baby's health. "She scolded me at every appointment that I should not be doing such hard exercise." Instead of accepting those admonishments to quit running, Shannon consulted a physician she'd gone to before moving to Puerto Rico. "He had actually studied exercise in pregnancy," she says, "and he was fine with what I was doing."

A DELIVERY ONLY AN ATHLETE COULD LOVE

With both of her children, Shannon went into labor right at 40 weeks. In her first delivery, she had to push for 3½ hours, a true athletic feat. After the baby was born, her doctor had to eat a bit of crow. "She admitted that I never would have been able to push that long if I hadn't been in shape," Shannon says. "This was the same doctor that had said I shouldn't be running, that I was going to have such a small baby."

The final triumph? A 7½-pound baby girl. (Her son, born 2½ years later, weighed over 8 pounds, and Shannon had run through that pregnancy, too.)

Shannon fit into her old clothes again within a week, so she didn't have much "baby fat" to lose. She could hardly wait to jump back into her old routine. "I had this herbal book that was my bible throughout pregnancy, and it suggested waiting until 8 weeks to exercise. I told myself I'd go 6, but at 4 weeks, I just couldn't handle it anymore."

Now that her kids are older, they understand why their dad wakes them in the mornings: Their mom is out doing something important. "I'm a better parent when I get exercise," she says. "When I don't, I'm crabby. It's hard to be a good mom when you're crabby."

SHANNON'S TIPS

Maintain your fitness routine. If you keep exercising when you're pregnant, your baby will just be "renting a room" and will move out with all her stuff when she's born.

Get a second opinion. If you're not satisfied with what your doctor tells you, seek further advice from a qualified health professional.

Maternity Miles

Whether you admit it or not, your running will change during pregnancy. At first those changes can be hard to get used to, but accepting them is the key to your success. Once you understand that you can't avoid a slower pace and fewer miles while you're pregnant, you can move ahead. "I consider myself a competitive athlete, and this was one time I could just really enjoy running," says Nora Tobin, an Anchorage runner and mother of two. "I didn't have a goal. Instead of thinking I had to train for a race, I thought about how much I liked being out there."

As your body gets bigger, you'll find that each mile takes longer, so don't clobber yourself trying to run as far as you used to. I coped with my newfound slowness by translating minutes into miles. For every 10 minutes I ran, I counted it as a "maternity mile." Since I started my pregnancy at an 8-minute pace and I finished it at an 11:30 pace, I figured that it evened out. Consider creating your own system for "maternity miles."

Snow provides extra cushioning for your heavy footfalls. For protection against the occasional slick spot, consider buying a pair of strap-on running cleats. Or try an inexpensive trick favored by Anchorage runners: Fasten about five or six ⅜-inch screws all the way into the treads of each shoe. (The screws are too short to poke through the soles of the shoes.) Make sure that the screws are evenly distributed so that you won't force your foot into a lopsided landing. Balance is already a challenge during pregnancy, so if your running paths become too icy, head for the treadmill or indoor track.

In extremely cold weather, stay within an easy walking distance of your house in case you injure yourself or simply get tired. Before your run confirm that someone can come to your rescue if necessary. (Carry a cell phone just in case.) Hypothermia rarely strikes a moving runner, but it's a different story if you stop—and these days you have to consider someone else. "Your body will try to protect the baby as much as it can, but not if it starts shutting down from hypothermia," says Debra Kristich-Miskill, a certified nurse-midwife in Anchorage.

Staying hydrated helps guard against hypothermia. Fill your water bottle with warm water to keep it from freezing. If carrying the water bottle makes your hand too cold, leave the bottle on your front step and circle around for it now and then. Or invest in a hydration system like a CamelBak and wear the "bladder" under your clothes. Cover exposed skin on your face and elsewhere with petroleum jelly to avoid frostbite.

Starting a Jogging Program Now That You're Pregnant

What if you've never run before—or haven't run in a while—and you want to start or restart a program now? Is it safe for you and your baby? Probably, assuming you have a low-risk pregnancy and you're willing to jog slowly and for short periods of time.

Until just a few years ago, doctors warned against starting any kind of brisk exercise program during pregnancy, but the latest research suggests it is safe. Always include your own doctor in your decision to exercise, and discuss it with her at each appointment: Your exercise program is an important component of your overall health profile. If your doctor tells you not to jog, don't—but do ask her to recommend another type of aerobic workout.

The best time to start an exercise program is at the beginning of the second trimester. "The discomforts of early pregnancy are starting to [ease]," says L. A. Wolfe, Ph.D., a professor of exercise physiology at the School of Physical Health and Education at Queen's University in Kingston, Ontario. "And it gives the baby a chance to get established. It makes sense not to do anything you're not used to in the first trimester."

Walking might be your best bet in the first trimester, especially if you've been completely sedentary. Work up to 30 minutes per session three or four times a week. After this becomes comfortable, gradually build up to jogging.

Start with an 8-minute walk followed by a slow 2-minute jog. Repeat twice for a 30-minute workout three or four times a week. When that begins to feel comfortable, decrease the walk to 7 minutes and

The Canadian Way

Do you need more specific advice on starting an exercise program while pregnant? Consider a set of guidelines most Canadian medical professionals provide to their pregnant patients. L. A. Wolfe, Ph.D., a professor of exercise physiology at the School of Physical Health and Education at Queen's University in Kingston, Ontario, and experts from the Canadian Society for Exercise Physiology created some recommendations after years of studying women who started an exercise program during pregnancy. The experts included the recommendations in an evaluation form called the Physical Activity Readiness Medical Examination for Pregnancy, or PARmed-X for Pregnancy. Although the form doesn't list jogging among the preferred types of exercise, many women use the guidelines for that purpose. With your doctor's blessing, you can use them, too.

The PARmed-X for Pregnancy suggests that pregnant women:

- Start their exercise program between the 14th and 28th week of pregnancy.
- Warm up and cool down for 10 to 15 minutes each session.
- Exercise for 15 to 30 minutes each session.
- Exercise three to five times per week.

The evaluation form advises women to monitor exertion in three different ways.

- Use the Borg Rating of Perceived Exertion.
- Try the "talk test." If you can easily carry on a conversation, you are exercising within safe limits.
- Stay within these target heart rate zones: 140 to 155 beats per minute if you are younger than age 20; 135 to 150 beats per minute if you are 20 to 29; 130 to 145 beats per minute if you are 30 to 39; and 125 to 140 beats per minute if you are 40 or older. (The American College of Obstetricians and Gynecologists eliminated all mention of heart rate limits from its most recent guidelines on exercise and pregnancy; however, Dr. Wolfe says that heart rate can be a valuable tool in conjunction with the RPE and talk test for new exercisers who begin their program after the first trimester.)

increase the slow jog to 3 minutes. Eventually you'll alternate 5 minutes of walking with 5 minutes of slow jogging.

When you're completely comfortable with this routine, you may begin jogging longer than you walk. Your goal is to work up to a 5- to 10-minute walking warmup, followed by 20 minutes of slow jogging, followed by a 5- to 10-minute cooldown.

Adapt this schedule to your own needs, and don't feel like you have to begin jogging just because the second trimester has started. Don't try to jog through any kind of pain: Walk home and call your doctor instead. If you are a detrained runner, don't talk yourself into believing you're more fit than you actually are. Running while pregnant is a new venture, and you must be a mother first and a runner second.

Never overexert yourself. If you feel out of breath (even if you haven't run as long as you'd planned), walk until you feel comfortable again. Remember the Borg Rating of Perceived Exertion—make sure you don't exceed 14. As you work out, drink from a water bottle or CamelBak to stay hydrated.

Finally, be prepared to find a comfortable pair of running shoes a half to a full size bigger than your regular shoe size because your feet expand with pregnancy. Ill-fitting shoes can cause problems, such as blisters or black toenails, and worn-down shoes can lead to back and knee pain.

CHAPTER 6

THE SECOND MONTH

SORE BREASTS AND SNUG SHORTS

IF YOU HELD A CROSS-COUNTRY RACE for 10 women in their second month of pregnancy, here's what might happen: Six would make it to the starting line, three would be at home throwing up, and one would be stuck in the Porta-Potty, constipated. All six at the starting line would stare bleary-eyed at you while they would wait for the gun to go off. One would cry (then laugh). Four would slog to the finish line, followed by one who'd stopped for a catnap and another holding a doughnut in each hand after a detour through the corner bakery. The only record set would be the number of no-shows.

> **PREGNANCY**
> **STEP**BY**STEP**
>
> Month 2: The image of your baby on the ultrasound leaves you dizzy with joy. First-trimester running—when your blood volume does not yet fill your expanding vascular system—also can leave you dizzy.

Pregnancy symptoms in month 2 can hit you in any number of ways. Your baby and your body are working in tandem to prepare for 7 to 8 more months of growth and development. The baby is about as big and heavy as a paper clip, but her heart is beating and her cells are dividing rapidly. Your body is creating a placenta to nourish her, and placenta-

91

building taxes your energy. Fatigue is nearly a guaranteed symptom at this stage of pregnancy.

FEELINGS AND SENSATIONS

Exhausted (Still)

Everyone tells you to take it easy now, get plenty of sleep, don't overdo it, and so forth and so on. It's all good advice, but what does it mean to a runner? Where is the balance between running and rest? Most runners who were interviewed for this book said that they forced themselves out the door, even when they felt tired. "The hardest part was getting myself to start. But I always felt good afterward," says Mcaire Trapp, a triathlete and mother of three from Winnetka, Illinois.

On the other hand, sometimes you have to let pregnancy take precedence over running. If you start running and your body stalls, walk instead. If walking drains you, go home and fluff up your pillow—it's time for a serious nap. Don't worry: Your unplanned rest does not mean that your fitness goals have gone out the window. In fact, "pregnancy is like armchair exercise," says Nancy Clark, R.D., nutrition counselor at SportsMedicine Associates in Brookline, Massachusetts, and author of *Nancy Clark's Sports Nutrition Guidebook.* "The body is already working very hard, so if you're too tired to go out and do purposeful exercise, don't fret about it." Some days your body works harder than other days, and you need to rest so that your body can do its job. Besides, the frustration you store up today will fuel your determination tomorrow.

Moody

You won't be mountain climbing and skydiving during pregnancy, but your emotions will. Thankfully, running can help straighten out your course. No scientific studies have connected endorphins with tranquility in pregnancy, but runners all seem to agree. "It was a bad situation for me if I didn't get out," says Diane Krapf, a Lake Forest, Illinois, runner and mother of two. "Running really relieved my stress."

"I felt good the whole day after running," says Kristin Alexander, a Chicago runner and mother of two. "Everything was changing and this was the one constant."

"Emotionally, exercise keeps you on an even keel, especially when your hormones are all out of whack," says Karen Cofsky, an athlete and mother of five from Oak Park, Illinois.

Sick to Your Stomach

If you're lucky, you will eke by with no morning sickness whatsoever. Morning sickness is a huge first-trimester complaint and, as illustrated earlier, can keep you from even making it to the starting line. If you don't feel the least bit nauseated, skip to the next section. The rest of you unlucky souls can keep reading.

Half of all pregnant women encounter some form of morning sickness, ranging from slight queasiness to frequent vomiting. If you're one of the 33 percent of pregnant women whose knees carve divots next to the commode, refrain from running until you start to feel better. "Running can aggravate your gastrointestinal tract and make it worse," says Patty Kulpa, M.D., a sports gynecologist in Gig Harbor, Washington. "And if you keep throwing up, you're going to get into electrolyte problems." This means dehydration. Staying hydrated can be tricky because drinking can sometimes trigger nausea. It may be difficult to take in very much liquid at a time, so try keeping a glass of water (or other inoffensive beverage) nearby, and sip every 10 to 15 minutes—whatever rate you can handle. Don't run if you feel dehydrated.

About 1 in 200 pregnant women develop a condition called *hyperemesis gravidarum*, which keeps you from holding down anything for weeks or months at a time and sometimes results in a lengthy hospital stay. Keep your doctor apprised of your ability to keep down food so that she can monitor you for this dangerous condition.

Beat the Morning Sickness Blues

The women who were interviewed for this book found creative ways to stop morning sickness from putting a dent in their running. Here are some of their suggestions.

- Eat a handful of saltine or graham crackers before getting out of bed.
- Eat small snacks every 2 hours instead of regular meals three times a day.
- Eat your food before drinking anything.
- Avoid strong smells, or breathe through your mouth if a smell is unavoidable.
- Pay attention to food aversions. If something makes you gag, don't force it on yourself.
- Drink peppermint tea, flat soda, or Gatorade.
- Suck on peppermint or ginger candy. One mother swore by wintergreen Life Savers to soothe her sour stomach.
- Wear an acupressure wristband (normally sold for seasickness), available in the pharmacy section of most discount stores.
- Stay hydrated as much as possible and drink liquid in small sips.

If you feel nauseated but don't tend to throw up, running is probably fine, although you should still discuss it with your doctor. Most women who were interviewed for this book ran through their queasiness or found a different time of day to run. "It was never morning sickness; more like an afternoon or night thing," says Alexander. "So I'd run first thing in the morning, just get up and go without having time to think about it."

"Sometimes my run was the only time of day when I didn't feel ill, especially during my first pregnancy, when I felt a low-grade nausea for 3 months," says Wendy Gellert, an Anchorage runner and mother of two.

Breast Tenderness

No one gets through pregnancy without major breast changes. In addition to the enlargement so obvious to everyone else, your breasts will almost certainly hurt. Rolling onto your stomach in bed, stepping into the shower spray, and pulling on and off your running bra may cause you to gasp.

Estrogen and progesterone are the culprits. These hormones begin their work early on to prepare your breasts for nursing. Although your bra size may continue to grow throughout your pregnancy, the sensitivity in your breasts and nipples should go away by the third or fourth month. In the meantime, find a running bra that provides maximum support and is easy to put on and take off.

Clumsy

You don't need a big belly to start losing your balance during pregnancy. You just need hormones. Your body begins to release the hormones relaxin and progesterone early in your pregnancy. They both help prepare your body for childbirth by loosening your joints and ligaments. In other words, they turn your body to rubber.

Pregnancy also induces a mental haze in most women, and the endorphins from running can compound the effect. Combat clumsiness by paying attention when you run. Don't zone out. Force yourself to locate the curbs, uneven grass, and potholes on your route. Be especially watchful for cars and bikes. If you feel you're becoming a danger to yourself and your baby, go to a local school and jog around the track.

A surprising number of pregnant women run on treadmills, which can be good for the joints—but hazardous to clumsy people. Run slowly and cautiously if you use a treadmill. The safest kind to use during pregnancy is the kind equipped with a magnetic key safety device. The key is linked to a cord that fastens to your clothing, so if you start to fall, the magnet pulls away from the treadmill and the machine stops. Barring this, look for a panic button (usually a big red button that says STOP) and train your hand to punch it in case you lose your balance.

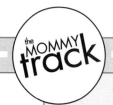

IRON MOM

Name: Geri Sorenson

Birth date: November 1964

Residence: Kildeer, Illinois

Occupation: Pharmaceutical sales manager

Children: Five; one singleton born 1995, followed by two sets of twins, born 1997 and 2000

BORN TO RUN

When Geri Sorenson joined the track team in second grade, she never guessed how far the sport would take her. She'd never heard of a marathon—little did she know that in adulthood she'd run at least 15 of them. "Running just seems to come naturally," she says.

"Geri was born to run," says Mcaire Trapp, her friend and fellow runner. The two ran the 1995 London Marathon together, finishing in a respectable 3:45. Geri was 29 weeks pregnant with her first child.

Geri concedes that marathons aren't for every pregnant runner. Her tip-top conditioning and a thumbs-up from her doctor allowed her to keep going. "My doctor told me, 'You can run the marathon, but promise me you'll drink a small bottle of water at every mile.'" Geri also promised to stop if anything hurt.

Later in that pregnancy, right around the 40-week mark, pain did interrupt her run. "Side stitches" slowed her to a walk a couple of times. Only after she'd gotten home, showered, and felt her water break did she understand what the pain really was.

During her second pregnancy—in which she carried twins—she cut back her weekly mileage from 60 to 40. At 32 weeks, she stopped running at the request of her doctor. "I didn't have any problems, but she was just uncomfortable with it. She'd never had a patient run with twins."

When pregnant for the third time—with another set of twins—she was able to run through 20 weeks. Then, because of a cerclage (a suture to hold the cervix closed that is a fairly common preventative measure for mothers of more than one set of multiples), her doctor urged her to quit running and switch to swimming instead. Geri's natural intensity kicked in. "I hated swimming, but I thought, 'If this is the only thing I can do, I'm going to make the most of it.'" She set her sights on training for the next Hawaii Ironman Triathlon. When she told her doctor about a 1½-mile swim session, he was not pleased. "He cut me off—told me to stop everything. He realized if he didn't, I would take it to the limit."

MAXIMIZING TRAINING TIME BETWEEN PREGNANCIES

Geri tucked in some major accomplishments between her three pregnancies. In 1999, before conceiving for the last time, she ran both a 50-mile and a 100-mile ultramarathon, placing second for women in the latter. She also started a tradition of pushing her kids in a triple stroller through the Chicago Marathon.

Even after she had to cut short her prenatal swimming, Geri continued to dream about the Hawaii Ironman. She now plans to make it a reality. "Just this week I got a training schedule together, and I'm taking some swimming instruction to make my strokes more efficient," she says. "It's just a matter of fitting it all in."

GERI'S TIPS

Stop before you get hurt. Never be too proud to stop running if your body hurts or if you're uncomfortable in any way. There's nothing negative about walking. It's a form of working out.

Get your head in the game. So much of running is psychological. After you deliver, don't force yourself to run if you're not mentally and physically ready. Run only when your head and body both feel good.

Go shoe shopping. Buy a brand new pair of running shoes soon after you deliver. It will help you psych up for your first run.

Falling Down

Over the years, I've had my share of Jerry Lewis moments. I've danced on top of my husband's toes, belly flopped while pushing my nephew on a swing, broken friends' dishes, and caused a host of other embarrassing incidents. So when I became pregnant, I had to be especially vigilant. My second pregnancy was during an icy winter, and I strapped on my running cleats every time I ventured out.

One day around week 7, I finished a slow 3-miler, breathed a sigh of relief, and then watched my legs fly out from under me. I landed on my wrist and thought that was the worst of my troubles. But when I undressed for my shower, I discovered blood in my underwear. The brownish spot was the circumference of a nickel. I placed a panicky call to my doctor's office, during which the triage nurse assured me that spotting after a fall or a hard workout (or even having sex) was normal at this point in my pregnancy.

I managed to stay vertical after that until month 7, when I tried to sneak downstairs carrying a load of books before my son woke up. Blinded by the books, I missed a step and skidded and bumped down our stairway on my side. This time the triage nurse made an emergency appointment to make sure that the placenta had not separated from my uterus and that the baby was not in distress.

The moral? Don't let down your guard. Remember that it's both easier to fall and potentially more serious later in the pregnancy. If you find yourself airborne, do what you can to avoid a belly landing. "Try to fall on your side or your buttocks," says Geralyn Coopersmith, C.S.C.S., exercise physiologist and owner of Physique Fitness in Ridgefield, Connecticut.

YOUR CONCERNS

Miscarriage

One of the things we fear most in early pregnancy is miscarrying the baby. Sadly, in the general population, the rate of miscarriage is around 15 to 20 percent. The good news is that several studies have shown that weight-bearing exercise (including running) does not increase a woman's risk of miscarriage.

If you have miscarried before, talk to your doctor before running while pregnant. In many cases it will still be fine for you to continue, but if a medical problem such as an incompetent cervix caused your previous miscarriage, you will most likely need to stop.

Overeating

If you're blessed with no morning sickness, you may find yourself veering in the other direction with an uncontrollable urge to gorge. Not only does your growing baby require more nutrients, but your body is generating hormones that make you want to eat more (and more and more . . .).

My friend Catherine Plichta, a Richmond, Virginia, runner and mother of two, is one of the most disciplined people I know. She laughs about gaining 40 to 50 pounds in both of her pregnancies. "The babies were always very low and out of the way, and I was able to consume amazing quantities of food."

When It's Not Okay to Run

The American College of Obstetricians and Gynecologists provides guidelines for situations in which a pregnant woman should not exercise. These include pregnancy-induced high blood pressure, symptoms and/or a history of preterm labor, vaginal bleeding, or premature rupture of membranes (broken water).

If you experience the following symptoms during and just after your run, stop and call your doctor: abdominal or low-back pain, vaginal bleeding, dizziness, faintness, increased shortness of breath, rapid heartbeat, difficulty walking, uterine contractions, chest pain, or fluid leaking from the vagina.

If you have a long-term disease or other medical problem, include your obstetrician and any other medical specialists you see in your decisions about running while pregnant. If they advise you not to run or exercise at all, listen to them. You have everything to gain and too much to lose.

Catherine's food odyssey lasted throughout her entire pregnancy both times. (She did lose the extra weight after her babies were born.) My own adventure tapered off soon after the first trimester ended, but not before I'd acquired some extra padding. I learned the hard way that even though pregnancy and running use extra calories, there is still such a thing as too much food.

Be honest with yourself, but don't sweat a spare pound or two. If you're paying attention to good nutrition and continuing to run, your pregnancy weight gain will likely stay within the 25- to 35-pound range that's considered healthy.

Constipation

By this month, you'll probably start to feel the metabolic effects of pregnancy. The progesterone in your body slows digestion, and slow digestion translates to harder feces. Add your iron-rich prenatal supplements to the mix and you have full-blown constipation.

Fortunately, running helps move the bowels—as anyone who's had runners' trots knows—as does eating extra fiber. With a few small dietary changes, you can work up to the recommended minimum of 25 grams a day. A peanut butter sandwich on whole grain bread can contain as much as 8 grams. (Learning to make a good peanut butter sandwich will come in handy someday, by the way.) A cup of lentil soup is worth 5 grams. Bran cereals contain up to 15 grams, and bran muffins can average between 3 and 8 grams.

If you're still constipated despite eating enough fiber, talk to your doctor. She may recommend that you take a fiber supplement like Metamucil or FiberCon or may suggest a stool softener. Just make sure that, when you go out for a run, you stay within sprinting distance of a bathroom.

Finally, drink enough fluids so that your urine is clear or very pale yellow. Staying hydrated won't magically rid you of constipation, but without hydration, you will almost surely suffer.

Note for Dads-to-Be

It's hard to anticipate how your mate will respond to the news of your pregnancy. Seems like you're never quite prepared for what he says—or doesn't say—especially after you've mentioned your plans to keep running. Here's a little icebreaker to open the channels of communication and get them flowing in the right direction. Feel free to photocopy it and lay it on top of his pillow.

Dear husbands and partners of pregnant runners:

Please accept my warmest congratulations on your baby on the way. I'm sure your wife's pregnancy has already been the source of much celebration. If she's the type to share details, you're undoubtedly learning more than you ever wanted to know.

Since your wife is a runner, you and she have additional concerns, the first being whether her exercise will harm the baby. Let me assure you, she has given this serious attention. There's a good chance she's already cleared it with her doctor, read books on exercise and pregnancy, and scanned the Internet for information. She understands that her body and the baby's are inextricably linked, and her job as a mother is to protect him or her.

So, what's your job? Some call it Chief Executive Supporter, some call it Assistant to the Queen. Mainly you're expected to listen well, empathize, agree, hold back opinions, and become slightly clairvoyant (my husband suggested I delete "slightly"). In short, you're expected to understand and support your wife, who may well have transformed into an eating, sleeping, scowling, bathroom-frequenting person you don't recognize.

Luckily, you can catch glimpses of her former self when she runs. Endorphins do wonderful things for pregnant women, especially when you consider the many other pleasures they've given up—alcohol, fashionable clothes, cappuccino.

That means it's in your best interest to encourage her running. Schedule a regular jog with her. Even if you're not a runner, you may be able to keep up with her slower pregnancy pace. If you are a runner, you may have to put in extra miles on your own and consider your run together your warmup or cooldown. Whatever you do, don't push her to run faster or farther than she feels comfortable. And if she doesn't feel like running—or quits altogether—respect her decision.

Pregnant husbands learn quickly to become nurturers—or to fake it. The more you learn now, the better off you'll be several months down the road. Believe it or not, someone even more demanding than your pregnant wife is just waiting to test your new skills.

Happy trails!

Chris

Two for the Price of One

The ultrasound shows twins. Should you keep running? If you have a healthy twin pregnancy and want to run, Dr. Kulpa recommends careful observation by your doctor. The fact is that twins are considered a high-risk pregnancy, she says. Women carrying twins are at greater risk for preeclampsia (also called *pregnancy-induced hypertension*), in which the placenta delivers insufficient oxygen and nutrients to the baby. They're also at risk for placental abruption, in which the placenta separates from the uterine wall. Premature labor is another danger, occurring in 20 to 50 percent of twin pregnancies. Running is out of the question when these health problems arise, and doctors generally prescribe bed rest or hospitalization.

Remember that being pregnant with twins will exhaust you more than if you're carrying just one baby. My friend Melissa David, a Winnetka, Illinois, runner and mother of three, describes her experience this way: "I remember being 3 months pregnant and getting exhausted just pushing my oldest child in the stroller for 30 minutes. I was absolutely not up for running. Sleep was my number one activity."

What about triplets or even more? Women with these kinds of multiple pregnancy are at even greater risk for all the problems described above. Doctors advise against vigorous exercise to avoid premature birth or other problems.

CHAPTER 7

THE THIRD MONTH

THE WORD IS OUT

BY THE END OF THIS MONTH, your baby will be about the size and weight of a fun-size candy bar. He graduates from embryo to fetus and begins to develop features like vocal cords and tear ducts (both of which he will use early and often after birth). A couple of your hormone-generated symptoms, like morning sickness and sore breasts, will be replaced by other, milder symptoms resulting from the baby's increased heft.

PREGNANCY STEPBY**STEP**

Month 3: Your running shoes feel tight as your feet expand and "grow." The baby's feet are forming toes.

FEELINGS AND SENSATIONS

Excited (and Defensive)

Since the threat of miscarriage decreases dramatically after the 12th week, many of us wait until the second trimester to tell family and friends about the pregnancy. As that time approaches, you may not be able to wait another 3 weeks to tell your closest family members. It's such a relief to share the big secret, especially when you know how excited they'll be. My husband barely got the words "We have news" out of his mouth before his mom cried, "Chris is pregnant!" My sister Anne sang "I get to be an aunt!" over and over into the phone.

It feels fantastic when other people share your joy. Unfortunately, some people will also share their opinions about your decision to run while pregnant—making you wish you'd kept the news to yourself. Thankfully, if anyone in my family thought I shouldn't be running, they stayed mum. Other women aren't so lucky. "I learned not to tell my mother," says Mcaire Trapp, triathlete and mother of three from Winnetka, Illinois. "She's often said my uterus is going to drop off."

Most people make such remarks to be helpful and probably don't realize that their comments are based upon outdated medical advice. Anticipate this kind of discussion and arm yourself with current information. The American College of Obstetricians and Gynecologists produces a handy little pamphlet called "Exercise During Pregnancy" and will send it to you free if you request it from their Web site. (See the Resource Guide.)

Better yet, don't allow yourself to get drawn into conversations with people who think they know better than you—your doctor being the rare exception.

Chunky

It's funny how you can see your baby in an ultrasound, suffer morning sickness, say "I'm pregnant" to a dozen family members and friends, and still not truly believe it. Here's the turning point: One day you'll bend over to tie your shoes and feel a croquet ball deep inside your belly. Just like that, you know *someone is in there*. This sensation usually happens around the 12th week. Along with it comes a feeling of dizziness—not from your sudden awareness, but because when you bend over, the baby momentarily cuts off your circulation. From here on, bending over becomes an exercise in hurrying to get the task done before you faint.

Clothing Note: Time to Go Prenatal

Since you've discovered the trials of bending over to tie your shoes, consider ordering some elastic laces that allow you to slip in and out of your running shoes. While you're at it, assess your shoes. Are your toes nipping at the ends? Some women's feet expand during pregnancy and require new shoes that are half a size to a full size larger.

It's not too early to decide what kind of reinforcement you want for your belly during running. Some women like support belts; other women claim these belts slip off. Maternity fitness clothing catalogs offer some excellent choices: Supportive shorts, tights, and unitards can all help reduce belly bounce. If you're not ready to spring for maternity clothes just yet, try wearing something already in your drawer like bike shorts, a tank swimsuit, or running tights. Another option: Buy a pair of compression shorts or tights a size or two larger than your regular ones. You'll use them again after delivery, before your body returns to its pre-pregnancy size.

Pregnancy encompasses your whole body. Your thighs get "pregnant," as do your butt, upper arms, and face. We won't even talk about your breasts. As your shape-hugging running clothes squeeze a little harder around your waist, cut yourself some slack. Do what it takes to mourn your runner's body. Have a good stare, cry if it helps, then move on. You'll reclaim your figure—or close to it—someday. The sacrifices you make in the meantime are well worth it.

Uncomfortable

You may already feel like your bladder is enrolled in a frequent fill-up program as you pay hourly visits to the bathroom. With pressure from the growing baby, these days your bladder may cause you more discomfort than ever. As with so many of the changes you experience during pregnancy, you simply have to grin and bear it. Things will improve sometime around the fourth month, when your uterus ascends into the abdominal cavity and vacates its cozy position up against your bladder.

To alleviate bladder discomfort during runs, limit your consumption of diuretic substances like cranberry juice and caffeine. Stop drinking all liquids an hour before you run, and make a pit stop just before you head out the door. If this is not your first pregnancy, you may experience minor stress incontinence. A light pad attached to your underwear will soak up any drips. Incontinence often can be prevented and/or eliminated with Kegel exercises, described in chapter 10.

YOUR CONCERNS

Fighting Minor Illness

Considering that pregnancy lasts almost a year, your chances of catching a cold, flu, or stomach virus are pretty good. Undoubtedly, your obstetrician has given you a list of approved medications (all three of them). Unfortunately, the list does not include anything laced with alcohol or other sleep aids. Instead of drugging yourself into a peaceful, pain-canceling slumber, you're limited to a decongestant, a mild pain reliever, and cough syrup, plus whatever home remedies you can patch together.

Then you have to decide whether or not to run. It's hard to imagine feeling so crummy and going through endorphin withdrawal on top of it. Respect that your body is growing a baby, building a placenta, and fighting illness. Take a few days off to let your body multitask.

If you have a fever, you definitely shouldn't run. An elevated body temperature (102.5°F or higher) may increase the risk of birth defects of the brain and spine, according to the March of Dimes. And if you can't keep food down, you're in danger of dehydration; running will only make it worse.

The good news is that, as a pregnant runner, you may be less likely to get sick in the first place. Here's why: Among nonpregnant athletes, several studies point to a temporary boost in immune function during and after exercise, which may have a cumulative effect against illness. The effect is reversed when athletes work out at higher intensities:

Inner Strength

When you're pregnant, you're not just growing another life inside your body. You're creating an entirely new organ, the sole purpose of which is to support that life. From conception through about week 14, your body builds a placenta, which delivers oxygen and nutrients to your baby. All you have to do is sit there.

Well, some people just sit there. Not you. You're outside staying fit, building muscle, and preparing your body to bounce back quickly after delivery. And that's not all. According to a 1995 study published in the journal *Placenta*, strenuous exercise enhances blood flow and helps build a bigger, better-functioning placenta. A regular-size placenta certainly will provide all the life support a baby needs under normal circumstances, but a stronger placenta will help protect the baby if the mother hemorrhages or encounters blood flow problems late in pregnancy. That's one more reason to get out for your run today.

Heavy exertion can suppress the immune system for up to a few days, which might explain why so many marathoners come down with colds and other minor illnesses soon after racing. Because your pregnancy forces you to slow down and run fewer miles, you may benefit from the positive influences on your immune system and dodge the bad ones.

Pregnancy normally suppresses the immune system and causes your colds and bouts with the flu to drag on, so take all the help you can get. If running keeps illness at bay in the first place, count it as yet another reason to lumber out the door every day.

Dealing with Injuries

If you weren't a runner, you might be oblivious to the hormone relaxin and its effects on your body. Most likely, your doctor mentioned it during your first conversation about running. As you read in chapter 6, beginning in the first trimester, relaxin loosens ligaments and softens cartilage in the pelvis and other areas of your body. As a result, pregnant athletes may be at higher risk for injury than nonpregnant athletes.

(continued on page 110)

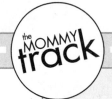

EXECUTIVE FITNESS

Name: Jill Bagley

Birth date: February 1961

Residence: Boulder, Colorado

Occupation: Human resources executive

Children: Two, born 1999 and 2002

FIT FOR MOTHERHOOD

"Fitness has always been a big part of my life," says Jill Bagley. Several years ago, when she traveled almost constantly on business, she tired of searching for a health club in every place she visited. Running became her workout of choice. Soon she was marathoning—completing six events before starting a family with her husband.

When she got pregnant the first time, Jill wasn't willing to let her fitness level slip. "I still enjoyed running and wasn't uncomfortable at all." Her doctor gave her the go-ahead to continue training, advising that as long as Jill could carry on a conversation throughout a run, the baby would get enough oxygen. Her loved ones, especially her husband, high-fived her efforts. "When I ran in the Bolder Boulder 10-K, my husband hung a BABY ON BOARD sign on my back," she says. "That drew a lot of positive comments and stories from the other runners."

In each of her pregnancies, Jill logged 25 to 30 miles a week throughout the first two trimesters, tapering a bit during the seventh month and finally switching over to cross-training when running became uncomfortable. She worked out on stairclimbers and cross-country ski machines and attended a sports fitness class that combined cardio and strength training.

Jill's two pregnancies were not markedly different, but the way she approached them was. "After the first pregnancy, it was fairly easy to get back into shape, so I was less concerned about it during round two," she says. "I was mellower and easier on myself the second time."

Both times, Jill delivered by C-section and then laid off running for 8 weeks. It took her only 3 weeks to get back to her low-impact gym workouts. "Because I had another form of exercise, I was okay with not running."

LATTE MILES

Now that life is back to "normal," how does a busy executive with two kids manage to run consistently? "I go out in the morning," she says. "If I don't do it then, it probably won't get done." Most days, Jill meets a running buddy at 6:00 for a "coffee run." That means running 6 to 7 miles through the foothills and canyons of Boulder, ending up at a coffee shop, and topping off with a latte. "It's great," she says. "You get your girlfriend time, you get your run in, and you get some coffee."

On weekends, she waits until the family wakes up, then puts her baby in the jogging stroller for the coffee run. "We do the same run up the hill, we stop for coffee, he sits in my lap and plays and sometimes has a bottle. Then I load him back up."

Jill is training for the Lake Tahoe Marathon, but she suffers from mother's angst. Her son's tolerance for the stroller goes only so far, so on long-run days she leaves him with his dad and sister. "I feel torn between spending time with my kids and focusing on running time for myself," she says. No doubt she'll find a way to make it all work.

JILL'S TIPS

Trust your instincts. Nobody knows your capabilities better than you do. Don't let anyone discourage you from running.

Get some belly support. Workout clothes that comfortably compress your belly are as much "head support" as anything, since they give you confidence that your baby isn't jostling around too much while you run.

Be prepared. When you take your baby with you on runs, carry a fully stocked diaper bag, your cell phone, and a front pack or other baby carrier in case your little one wants out of the stroller.

Pregnancy also creates certain musculoskeletal changes that can contribute to injuries. By the end of 9 months, for example, you will have added between 25 and 35 pounds to your frame, undergone a forward pelvic shift, experienced a curve in your lower back and rounding in your upper back, and adapted all the muscles in your legs and torso to accommodate your new shape. It's only natural that your running gait changes, too. This means that your feet strike the ground in an entirely new way than they always have. Sometimes those differences can create pain. The following pains, strains, and injuries are common to pregnant runners. Treat them with the suggestions here and turn back to chapter 3 for stretching and strengthening exercises that will counteract them.

Plantar fasciitis: The plantar fascia is the connective tissue that runs along the bottom of your foot between the heel bone and the base of your toes, and when it tears—ouch! The pain starts in the heel and radiates through your foot. Here's how it happens: When women run, they pronate—the arches collapse and roll inward—more than men do. During pregnancy, pronation gets worse as your pelvis expands and your knees turn slightly inward. (Think of your legs making an hourglass shape and you'll get the picture.)

Treat it by resting, icing, massaging your foot (but not the tender area), and lightly stretching your calves. When you're not pregnant or breastfeeding, it's fine to treat it with anti-inflammatory medication like ibuprofen. Until then, find shoe inserts that support your arches. You can purchase them at most running specialty shops and athletic equipment stores. If the problem persists, stop running and see a physical therapist, sports medicine physician, or podiatrist.

Strengthening your deep hip musculature with functional squat exercises may also help, since many of the leg and foot alignment problems that pregnant women have originate in the hip area.

Runner's knee: Poor alignment in the hips, legs, and feet during pregnancy also contribute to runner's knee, which occurs when the kneecap starts to slip out of its groove in the femur (thigh bone) and bone grinds against bone. Runner's knee starts as a pain behind and surrounding the kneecap. In extreme cases, a person with runner's knee will notice swelling around the knee and should stop running and see a sports medicine physician.

Treat runner's knee by using a compression sleeve that has a hole for your knee, icing tender areas around the knee, and stretching and strengthening your hips, quads, and hamstrings.

Hip problems: The changes in your posture and the loosening ligaments in your pelvis can cause a number of hip problems during pregnancy, including referred pain that travels to your groin, your knees, and even your feet. If you suspect hip problems, don't try to diagnose them yourself. Ask your doctor to refer you to a sports medicine physician or physical therapist.

Pubic pain: You can't miss it—a sudden, sharp twinge in your pubic area that's impossible to ignore. The pain can strike anytime, anywhere, and it can make a simple movement like rolling over in bed excruciating. Here's what's happening: Your pubic bone is situated front and center in your pelvis, right between your legs. It's held together by connective tissue called the *pubic symphysis*, which widens throughout your pregnancy in preparation for childbirth. During this transitional time it can become irritated. Running and other high-impact exercise only exacerbate the irritation.

Call your obstetrician immediately if you feel this sharp pain, and don't try to run. After you've been examined—and if the pain goes away—you may be able to resume some low-impact exercise that your doctor or physical therapist approves.

Round-ligament pain: The round ligament attaches the uterus to the labia majora. Your growing uterus stretches this ligament, creating a pulling (and sometimes painful) sensation in the pelvis. Unless the pain is persistent, you don't have to do anything. Add more belly support and mention it to your doctor.

Back pain: Most back pain results from looseness in your ligaments and/or the weight of your growing baby. Remember the "S"

RICE to the Rescue

The RICE treatment—rest, ice, compression, elevation—is a noninvasive, highly effective method of dealing with an injury. "For the garden-variety musculoskeletal injury, RICE is always the best first line of defense," says Geralyn Coopersmith, C.S.C.S., exercise physiologist and owner of Physique Fitness in Ridgefield, Connecticut. "It goes a long way toward preventing swelling and inflammation." As a pregnant runner, you'll want to get to know the RICE treatment well, since pregnancy limits the kind of pain medication you might normally use.

Here's how to do it.

Rest: Stay off the injury as much as possible, and cross-train with exercise that doesn't cause more pain.

Ice: Use anything cold—a bag of frozen vegetables, an ice pack, or a zipper bag full of ice cubes. Coopersmith has even used a cold can of soda in a pinch. Always wrap the injured area in a couple of layers of plastic wrap, a wet towel, or an elastic bandage to protect your skin. Ice your injury for 10 to 15 minutes on, 10 to 15 minutes off, for as many cycles as you can throughout the day.

Compression: Wrap the area with an elastic bandage. The compression will help keep swelling down. Make sure the bandage isn't too tight; loosen it if you feel pain or numbness in the area.

Elevation: Raise the injured area to reduce swelling.

curve I mentioned in chapter 3? "The lower back becomes more arched and the upper back becomes more rounded," says Joy Backstrum, a physical therapist in Anchorage, Alaska. If lower-back pain radiates into your legs or you have any other persistent back pain, talk to your doctor. She may prescribe exercises or a trip to a sports medicine physician or physical therapist.

Traveling with Baby on Board

Flying during a low-risk pregnancy should be no problem, as long as you're under 36 weeks or under 35 weeks along for international trips, according to the American College of Obstetricians and Gynecologists. If you need to travel later in your pregnancy, consult your obstetrician. Contact the airline beforehand to check their policy about pregnant passengers. Some airlines require a note from your doctor— signed within 72 hours of your trip—stating that your pregnancy is low-risk and establishing your due date. Driving to your destination should also be no problem, but use extra caution for the baby's sake and your own. As you approach your due date, stay within a 1- to 2-hour drive of your preferred hospital. Whether traveling by air or by car, always wear a seatbelt. Tuck it under your bulging belly instead of over it.

Travel won't put a dent in your running plans if you plan well. For starters, add these items to your packing list as needed.

- Water bottle

- Plastic zipper bags (to fill with ice for sore spots or injuries)

- Small plastic bottle of fabric wash in case you need to launder your running clothes in the sink

- Sanitary pads (if your bladder has been leaky)

- Sunblock

- Rain gear, hats, mittens, and extra layers for cold climates

- Fanny pack, assuming it still fits around your waist, or a hand-carried bag containing your picture identification, insurance card (in case of premature labor or injury), cell phone or coins for a pay phone, local emergency phone numbers, and cash for a cab ride back to your accommodations

If you're staying in a hotel by yourself, ask the front-desk clerk or concierge where it's safe and unsafe to run. Mention where you're going and when you plan to be back. Tuck your key in to your pocket or bag to avoid advertising yourself as an out-of-towner.

While running in unfamiliar territory, stay alert. Don't jaywalk. Traffic patterns are probably different from what you're used to, especially if you're in a different state or country. Remember that endorphins can make you loopy, and if you're experiencing the mind fog that sometimes accompanies pregnancy, you can get lost if you don't pay attention.

As a pregnant runner, you stand out from the crowd. Even if you're in a seemingly safe area, watch the people around you. "Be alert. Be aware of the environment. If people are loitering on a corner, don't run by them. Change your route if you have to," says Paul Henry Danylewich, director of White Tiger Street Defense in Montreal, Quebec.

For runners, one of the hardest things about traveling—even when you're not pregnant—is squeezing runs into an altered schedule. For one thing, your high-energy period will change with the time zones, so you will need to either move your regular running slot to a more suitable time of day or endure some lackluster runs until you adjust. And you often have to accommodate more people than at home. Let your traveling companions or hosts know ahead of time that you plan to run. Find out which times of the day will be least disruptive to them. Then choose a time slot for running and stick to it.

PART 3:
THE SECOND TRIMESTER

CHAPTER 8

THE FOURTH MONTH

WELCOME TO THE HONEYMOON

IF YOU'VE NEVER BEEN PREGNANT BEFORE, it's hard to imagine how it feels. For a close approximation, picture a bowling ball or a gallon jug of water resting on your belly. What would it be like with that on the inside, pressing its weight directly onto your organs? How's that going to feel when you're running?

PREGNANCY STEPBYSTEP

Month 4: You enjoyed a sweaty 5-miler today. Your baby has developed sweat glands on the palms of her hands and soles of her feet.

"It was the heaviness that felt different," says Leanne Molinero, an Australian runner and mother of two. "There was a lot of pressure on my pelvis, and I could feel the baby's weight pulling down on my abdomen." Others describe the heaviness as making them feel sluggish. Later in the pregnancy, the growing baby may widen your stance and give your stride a side-to-side motion, like a speed skater minus the skates—and the speed.

As you enter your second trimester, your feelings and concerns change right along with your growing girth. Here's how to take them in stride.

FEELINGS AND SENSATIONS

A Little Closer to Normal

Some people call the second trimester the honeymoon phase of pregnancy. Although there's nothing romantic about your emerging belly or the fact that you've stopped throwing up, you'll probably like this time in your pregnancy. You'll find more energy, become breathless less often, and feel less queasy. When you run, you may even forget you're pregnant for a while.

For me, the second trimester in both my pregnancies was clearly marked. My running tights left indentations on my belly, and within a very short time I had to switch to maternity clothes. Over the course of those 3 months I began "filling out" my maternity clothes, and by the end there could be no doubt in anyone's mind about my prenatal status.

And it's no wonder. During that 90-day period the baby snowballs from a 1-ounce, 3-inch-long peewee to a 2-pound, foot-long child. She goes from being utterly dependent on your body to having a good chance of surviving a premature delivery.

As long as you don't mind doing laundry, just a handful of new clothes will see you through the bulk of your pregnant running. The rest can come from your (or your husband's) closet. If you do purchase new clothes, buy as you grow. (The Resource Guide lists retailers that offer maternity workout clothes.)

When buying, concentrate on supporting your belly and breasts. This may sound obvious, but some workout clothing merely covers your belly—and does nothing to secure it. Look for shorts, tights, or unitards that compress the pregnant belly and hold it in place. Many manufacturers also offer a broad selection of maternity workout shirts to loosely cover your expanding midsection and wick away sweat.

Make sure your shoes still have some spring left in the soles. If you've put more than 300 miles on them, it's time for a new pair. "If a pregnant runner works out with bad shoes, she may develop pain in her back or in her knees," says Patty Kulpa, M.D., a sports gynecologist from Gig Harbor, Washington. Invest in bigger shoes if you find your feet swelling or otherwise expanding during pregnancy.

Exercise bras are a more personal choice. During the first month or two of pregnancy, you can continue to wear your regular running bras, and some women won't need to replace them during pregnancy. But if your breasts bounce too much or feel constricted, start shopping around.

Simply graduating to a larger size in the bra you already wear often helps. If your breast shape also changes, you might have to retire your favorite style and start from scratch.

> ## How to Find Big Stuff Cheap
>
> Several runners interviewed for this book did not buy a stitch of maternity workout wear. Instead, they:
>
> • Wore two of their regular running bras at a time for extra support
>
> • Wore the extra-large race T-shirts they had collected during the year leading up to their pregnancies
>
> • "Borrowed" their husband's compression shorts (and replaced them later)
>
> • Wore a one-piece swimsuit or leotard as a maternity unitard underneath a pair of baggy shorts and a T-shirt

Here are some tips for reentering the running-bra search.

• If your enlarged breasts are still in the A-, B-, or C-cup range, you can use a compression-type bra that simply restrains the breasts. If your breasts have expanded into the D range or beyond (did you know bras come in size G?), you may need an encapsulation bra that isolates each breast in a separate cup.

• If your breasts are in the smaller range (A, B, or C cup), try to find a bra that slips over your head and has no "hardware"—snaps, zippers, hooks, and eyes. If you are larger-breasted, pulling a bra over your chest can be difficult, especially when you remove it after a sweaty

(continued on page 122)

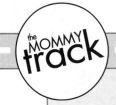

MARATHON MOM

Name: Lynda Del Missier

Birth date: June 1965

Residence: Tampa, Florida

Occupation: Stay-at-home mom

Children: Two, born 1997 and 2000

A RUNNING PURIST

Lynda Del Missier loves running. Just running. She wants nothing to do with stairclimbers or elliptical trainers. She hates weights. After her kids were born, she hired a personal trainer but ended up regretting it. "I thought, 'Why am I paying him all this money when I can put on my running shoes and get outside?'" she says.

Lynda's love of running carried her through two pregnancies. She didn't alter her mileage, but she did slow down, managing to run until the end of the sixth month during the first pregnancy. "I live in Florida, and it's hotter than hell," she says. That meant running in the early mornings and carrying water on even her shortest runs.

After having her first child, Linda remained undaunted by motherhood and decided to pursue one of her long-standing goals: the marathon.

PUTTING ASIDE A GOAL

As Lynda logged mile after mile of rigorous training, she realized that something didn't feel right. Her long runs of 15 miles exhausted her far more than she'd expected. And she felt weak and sick to her stomach most of the time. The symptoms landed her in the doctor's office, where she was asked if pregnancy was a possibility. *There's no way,* she remembers thinking. *I cannot be pregnant.*

Once the doctor confirmed that a baby was in fact on the way, a hopeful Lynda asked whether she could still run the marathon for which she'd been training so hard. He told her to go ahead but to always run slowly enough that she could still talk. To be extra safe, Linda wore a heart rate monitor and kept her rate within a prescribed range as she trained.

Nevertheless, the heavy mileage proved too much. "I was exhausted," she says. She decided to focus on a half-marathon instead.

In the end, her body had different plans. Around the time she decided to cut back, she was diagnosed with placenta previa, a potentially dangerous condition in which the placenta touches or blocks the cervix. In the span of a few weeks, she'd gone from marathon training to complete bed rest. "It was the pits," she recalls.

TAKING HER TIME

After both births, despite longing to lace up again, Linda waited a full 3 months before running. She worried about coordinating breastfeeding with running, and wondered whether exercise would decrease her milk production. By the time she did run again, her body had healed completely and breastfeeding was firmly established. "I started doing a little walking and then I'd walk-run and then I slowly got back into it."

Now Lynda runs with two other moms. "We go at 6:00 in the morning, even on weekends," she says. "When we're done, our kids are just waking up."

Lynda is thinking marathon again these days. She's already completed a half-marathon and she plans to run another soon. When her younger child starts kindergarten, she'll ramp up her mileage and reach again for the goal she came so close to once before.

LYNDA'S TIPS

Forget about the pounds. "If you're weight conscious, you may feel discouraged when the scale continues to go up despite your exercise. But this is the one time gaining weight is okay."

Choose a heart rate monitor carefully. "I bought one that chafed me raw during my long runs. I still have the scar."

Have patience. "It's the hardest part, but you have to be patient and not push yourself too hard. You'll get there."

run. You will probably need a bra that opens, making hardware unavoidable. Check that the hardware does not touch your skin, or gouging may result.

- Look for wide-backed bras to give you more frontal support. Some maternity workout bras have special panels across the upper back.

- Avoid bras that creep under your arms. They often chafe the tender skin.

- Run in place in the dressing room to see how the bra feels.

- Stretch your arms up and swing them in circles. If the bra rides up or becomes uncomfortable, it probably won't work for you.

Fetal Movement

One of the very best things about the second trimester is that you'll start to feel your baby move. Sometime between the 14th and 26th week, you'll feel a sensation different from anything you've ever experienced. A ripple will pass through your lower abdomen, one you know your body didn't create. When you place your hand on your tummy, your palm and fingers will press against something rock hard. Then you'll grab your husband's hand as soon as it is within reach. (A well-trained husband learns to ooh and ah right along with you, even when he can't distinguish the baby's movements from yours.) Thereafter, you'll find your hand flying to your belly every time you feel movement.

During both my pregnancies, I loved to lie in bed with my hand on my abdomen before I fell asleep. My first son seemed to roll and stretch inside the womb, as though he was just waking up from a long nap. My second son found a way to do Tae Bo in there. Not surprisingly, the first was born mellow and the second anything but.

When you run, the baby's heart rate goes up, too. Even so, she'll probably stay very quiet throughout your run. Within a few minutes after you've stopped, she'll begin to move again. Although it's not necessary, you may take comfort in counting your baby's movements after each workout. Ten fetal movements or more in 1 hour is a good indicator that the baby is doing fine. If your baby does not seem to move at all, lie down on your left side, drink fluids, and call the doctor. She'll probably want to see you for an evaluation.

Gassy

Some women liken the sensation of fetal movement to gas pains. The difference is that the gas you're feeling these days can be downright unpleasant. "Progesterone slows down bowel transport time," says Jan Whitefield, M.D., an Anchorage obstetrician. Not only does that mean you're constipated and gassy, but your bowel might deceive you into thinking you're having labor pains. Gas cramps can radiate from low in your pelvis all the way around to your back, creating a girdle of pain. If you feel discomfort like this, stop and walk. Gas pains usually resolve themselves. If they don't go away—or they get worse— walk home and call the doctor.

You'll probably feel the "gas girdle" more frequently as your pregnancy progresses. And your increasingly compressed bowels may even give you confusing signals. "The problem I had from the get-go was abdominal distress," says Lisa Keller, an Anchorage triathlete and mother of two. "I was constipated during both pregnancies. I felt like I had to poop the whole run, then I'd get home and couldn't do it."

YOUR CONCERNS

Early Contractions

You'll learn the term *Braxton-Hicks contraction* later in your pregnancy when you're trying to tell the difference between pre-labor and the real thing. Braxton-Hicks contractions make you feel like your baby is squeezing into a little ball inside your abdomen. They don't hurt—they just make your belly feel peculiar for a while.

It is important to learn the difference between a Braxton-Hicks contraction and a labor contraction. In addition to not causing pain, the

Braxton-Hicks variety stays in the middle to upper portion of your abdomen. True labor contractions feel an awful lot like menstrual cramps and originate in your lower back, radiating around front. It goes without saying, however, that if you feel a twinge in your pelvis but don't know how to identify it, call your doctor.

Beginning in the second trimester, athletes frequently notice a Braxton-Hicks contraction at the beginning of each exercise session. "You'll become more sensitive to it as you get further along in your pregnancy, unless you've already had kids," says Dr. Kulpa. "In that case, you'll pick it up a lot sooner." The sensation should disappear within a minute or two. But if you feel as many as four of these within 1 hour, go home, drink fluids to make sure you're hydrated, and lie down on your side. Call your doctor if you feel the squeezing sensation on and off for 20 minutes or more. Braxton-Hicks contractions could start dilating and effacing your uterus in preparation for a premature birth.

Anemia

One of the more serious "side effects" of second-trimester pregnancy is anemia. It usually strikes between the fourth and sixth months as your blood volume expands and the baby grows bigger and demands more from you nutritionally. As a result, your iron stores become depleted, making you feel sluggish and tired, especially when you run. That first-trimester breathlessness you thought was gone now makes an unwelcome comeback.

Your doctor will check for anemia at your first prenatal visit and again around the 20th week. If you feel like some of your first-trimester woes are returning, ask to be tested ahead of schedule. Your low iron stores won't hurt the baby, but your running will suffer.

Anemia is usually treated with iron supplements and a change in diet. Iron-rich foods include beef, shrimp, spinach, refried beans, turkey, prune juice, and fortified breakfast cereal. Your body will not absorb the iron in fortified cereals well, but adding vitamin C–packed juices or fruits to your meals will help with absorption. Remember that all that iron in your diet can cause constipation, so drink lots of liquids and eat fiber-rich veggies, fruits, whole grains, and legumes.

Nasal Congestion

Exercising during pregnancy can be a double-hankie affair. Your legs aren't the only things running. Higher levels of estrogen and progesterone increase blood flow everywhere—including your nasal passages. They tend to swell and get softer, making you stuffy and prone to nosebleeds. (Your gums may also bleed when you brush your teeth.) Bring handkerchiefs or tissues on each run, and don't be surprised if a little blood comes out when you blow.

Your Evolving Anatomy

In this book we focus mostly on obvious body parts—the ones you see and think about each time you run. But your internal baby-building system is also part of the equation. Here's a primer on running and your prenatal anatomy.

Placenta: What a coincidence that the placenta, which provides oxygen and food to your baby, is shaped like a dinner plate. The placenta also processes waste from the baby, creates pregnancy hormones, and screens out many harmful substances. This disposable organ attaches to the inside of your uterine wall and connects your blood supply to the baby's through the umbilical cord. The placenta will weigh a pound or more by the time you expel it from your body after the baby's birth. As long as your placenta is healthy and well-positioned, running will help it grow and function better.

Umbilical cord: This lifeline connecting you and your baby is made up of three blood vessels wrapped in protective tissue. One vessel is a vein that brings blood loaded with oxygen and nutrients from the placenta to your baby. The other two are arteries that haul waste products away from baby to the placenta. At 28 weeks' gestation, the umbilical cord reaches a full 22 inches long. At least two studies suggest exercise will not harm umbilical cord function. However, if an

(continued on page 128)

Pregnancy Problems You Need to Understand

Most pregnancy-related illnesses crop up in the second or third trimester. Being familiar with the symptoms—and knowing whether you can still run—will help you take the best care of your baby and yourself.

CONDITION	WHAT IT IS	CAUSE
Gestational diabetes	Pregnancy-generated diabetes	Your pregnant body interferes with insulin (the substance that processes glucose in your body) to guarantee the baby a large glucose supply. Sometimes too much glucose begins circulating in your bloodstream. In a normal pregnancy, your body will add more insulin to process the glucose, but when you have gestational diabetes, you cannot produce enough insulin or your body cannot use the insulin it does make
Preeclampsia (a.k.a. toxemia, pregnancy-induced hypertension)	High blood pressure occurring during pregnancy	Unknown
Placenta previa	A low-lying placenta that touches (or blocks) the internal opening of the cervix. Placenta previa can cause excessive bleeding during delivery, and if the placenta blocks the cervix, vaginal delivery will not be possible	Unknown, although risk is higher in smokers and women with uterine scarring
Placental abruption (abruptio placentae)	A placenta that separates from the uterine wall in part or whole before delivery	Unknown, but risk is higher in women who smoke, are pregnant with multiples, have an abnormal uterus or umbilical cord, experience high blood pressure, or have suffered abdominal trauma (such as in a car accident or abuse)

If you suspect something is wrong with your pregnancy, contact your doctor immediately.

SYMPTOMS	WHEN DIAGNOSED	TREATMENT	CAN YOU RUN?
Sugar in the urine, revealed during your monthly urine test at the doctor's office; excessive thirst; excessive urination; increase in blood pressure. Often the pregnant woman doesn't notice any symptoms	In most cases, gestational diabetes is discovered during a routine screening test at your obstetrician's office between the 24th and 28th weeks	Change in diet and occasionally insulin injections	Yes, with your doctor's permission. Exercise is almost always recommended for women with gestational diabetes
May experience some or all: high blood pressure, protein in the urine, sudden swelling of hands and face, excessive weight gain (as much as 1 pound a day), blurred vision, severe headaches, stomach pains	Anytime during the pregnancy	Bed rest and sometimes drugs to prevent convulsions. If the baby is close to term, the doctor will likely induce labor. Left untreated, it could progress to eclampsia, in which the mother suffers from convulsions and coma, putting the baby's life in danger if not delivered quickly.	No
Bright red blood that may stop and start; sometimes no symptoms	After 20 weeks' gestation. (A low-lying placenta discovered before 20 weeks may move upward as the uterus stretches)	Reduced activity; sometimes bed rest or hospitalization	No
Vaginal bleeding, sometimes accompanied by a tender abdomen and abdominal pain	20 weeks or later; most often in the third trimester	Hospitalization. If the baby is near term (37 weeks), she will probably be delivered early	No

(continued)

Pregnancy Problems You Need to Understand (cont.)

CONDITION	WHAT IT IS	CAUSE
Premature rupture of membranes	A hole in the amniotic sac that allows amniotic fluid to leak	Unknown
Thrombophlebitis and deep venous thrombosis	A blood clot in a vein of the leg (or less commonly an arm). When a clot is in veins near the skin, it's called *thrombophlebitis*; the biggest risks associated with it are infection and damage to the vein. Deep venous thrombosis occurs deeper in the veins and is more serious because a clot may break off and lodge in the brain, heart, or lungs	The body increases its clotting mechanism in preparation for the bleeding that occurs during delivery. Risk factors include varicose veins, anemia, being over age 30, a history of clots, being overweight, entering your fourth (or greater) pregnancy, being sedentary, and bed rest

ultrasound indicates that your umbilical cord is abnormal, your doctor may advise you not to run.

Womb: When you became pregnant, you probably started thinking differently about your uterus. Instead of being the source of your monthly woes, it now serves as someone's home. When you run or do other rhythmic exercise, your baby may feel it as a gentle rocking motion. Running and other exercise should have no effect, unless your uterus is abnormally structured (which could be discovered during an ultrasound or after you've had a previous miscarriage or premature delivery). In this case, your doctor may recommend limiting activity to keep you from early labor.

Amniotic fluid: Amniotic fluid is truly a multipurpose solution. It cushions your baby and cycles through her body to promote the de-

SYMPTOMS	WHEN DIAGNOSED	TREATMENT	CAN YOU RUN?
Fluid gushing or trickling from the vagina that usually gets worse when the mother is lying down	Second or third trimester	Hospitalization and antibiotics. Occasionally the rupture heals by itself and the mother can return home. If the baby is at term, the doctor will deliver early	No
A tender, red area on the thigh or calf, pain and heaviness in one leg, distension of veins in one leg, swelling in one leg, fever	Anytime during pregnancy, labor, and delivery; and most commonly in the first 6 months postpartum	Varies based on severity; rest, elevation of the leg, moist heat, topical medication, compression stockings, and anticoagulant drugs. Running may help prevent future clots	Thrombophlebitis usually clears up within 2 weeks, and your doctor may allow you to run. With deep venous thrombosis, you most likely will not be allowed to run

velopment of her lungs and gastrointestinal tract. Amniotic fluid allows the baby to move around, enabling her muscles and bones to develop normally—much the way running enhances your muscles and bones. To keep amniotic fluid at a healthy level, stay hydrated before, during, and after your runs.

Amniotic sac: Poetically known as your *bag of waters* and less poetically as *membranes*, your amniotic sac surrounds the baby and contains the amniotic fluid. If the amniotic sac ruptures prematurely (before 37 weeks' gestation), you will not be allowed to run until after delivery. (If it ruptures at term, your labor has begun or most likely will be induced within 24 hours.) Running with this condition could cause compression of the umbilical cord, which could be deadly for your baby. Bed rest is likely. The good news is that exercise will not *cause* a healthy amniotic sac to rupture.

Some women have a medical condition that causes them to have too much or too little amniotic fluid. Doctors often prescribe bed rest for such problems.

Cervix: As you get closer to your due date, your cervix will command a lot of your attention. If you didn't know better, you might think it is a stand-alone organ rather than simply the "neck" of your uterus. The cervix's job is to stay tightly shut until labor day (or just prior), at which point it slowly opens to allow your baby through. If it begins to open (dilate) and/or thin out (efface) before 37 weeks, your doctor will advise you to curtail your activity level and may even put you on bed rest.

CHAPTER 9

THE FIFTH MONTH

YOU AND THE BUDDHA

"I HATE THE FIFTH MONTH," my friend Meg confided during her second pregnancy. "You're showing just enough that everyone thinks you're fat." This was true for her and for other tallish people with ample room in their abdominal cavity. The rest of us started looking fat way back in the fourth month. Fortunately, this in-between time doesn't last long. Your Buddha belly will fill out the round seams of your maternity clothes in 3 or 4 more weeks. In the meantime, you should try to enjoy some of the best, most comfortable running of your pregnancy.

> **PREGNANCY STEP**BY**STEP**
>
> Month 5: Your baby seems to have a sense of humor. When you run, he stays completely still; when you lie down for a nap, he begins exercising.

FEELINGS AND SENSATIONS

Energetic

Everyone encouraged you to take naps during the first trimester when your body was begging you to rest. And resting is just as important now, when your energy levels are naturally higher and you're more inclined to overdo it on the road. For each medium to hard day of running, give yourself an easy day in which you jog slowly, do a run-walk combination, cross-train lightly, or rest. "You've got to have balance," says Patty Kulpa, M.D., a sports gynecologist in Gig Harbor, Washington. "Otherwise the baby's not going to grow, and you're going to be at a higher risk for making mistakes and injuring yourself."

When you can, spend time relaxing after your runs. Sometimes extra rest will be impossible, but sneak it in whenever you find a pocket of time. Take a long bath, read a book, watch a movie, phone your best friend, or just stare at the wall. If you run before work or on

Coping with Concerned Citizens

Eventually your pregnancy becomes obvious, especially if you wear form-fitting workout clothes. People will begin to stare. Even in our modern times, a pregnant runner is an unusual sight. A car passes and the driver cranes her neck to check out your belly. Pedestrians eye you in their peripheral vision. After a few weeks, people you've never noticed before will start saying "Hi" as if they know you.

Then come the comments—mostly the high-five, you-go-girl variety. If you're the kind of person who runs faster at races when people cheer for you, you'll eat up these comments and harvest an extra boost of energy from them. Write down the praise in your running journal and review it next time you need motivation to get out the door.

The other type of remark you may hear is the Concerned Citizen variety. "A couple of times when I was on the treadmill at the gym, women came up to me and said, 'I really don't think you should be running,'" says Lisa Keller, an Anchorage triathlete and mother of two. "I'd just tell them to give me a break."

Although you may never need it, it's handy to line up a response to lob back at Concerned Citizens. My favorite (though I never got to use it) is: "My obstetrician is fine with my running. Are you an obstetrician?" Better yet, you can always pretend you're not pregnant and that they've just insulted you. If a Concerned Citizen persists, ignore him or her and move on. Most likely you're being baited into a no-win argument.

your lunch hour, kick back as soon as you get home in the evening. Your well-rested body will help you run far into your pregnancy.

Out of Shape

Illness, injury, or the rigors of pregnancy may force you into a short layoff period. A layoff period is a time during which you do not run at all. It can last from a few days to a few months, and how you return to running will depend on how long your layoff period was. It takes 3 weeks to lose most, if not all, of your fitness level. If a head cold has kept you inactive for 4 or 5 days, you may be able to pick up where you left off. But if you stopped running during 2 months of morning sickness, you will need to train like a new runner.

Itchy

Someday, when women take another step in evolution, I hope we get a secret storehouse of skin to add to our pregnant bellies. Until that time, our poor skin has to stretch to astounding lengths to cover the baby and all his cushioning. That makes us itch. (Sweaty running tights don't improve the situation.) Keep your belly moisturized, and try calamine lotion on especially itchy days.

Heartburn

Heartburn comes to call just about the time your other unwelcome guest—morning sickness—has finally taken leave. It happens because the baby is big enough to be squeezing your stomach and nudging its juices into your esophagus. Pregnancy hormones are also to blame for your discomfort; these hormones relax the muscle tissue that would normally keep food and acids in your stomach, where they belong. Though running can aggravate heartburn, it doesn't cause any harm.

"I could eat anything—a banana, even—and my stomach would give me such bad heartburn," says Wendy Gellert, an Anchorage runner and mother of two. Her doctor recommended an over-the-counter antacid, which helped. Banana-induced heartburn is less common than, say, pepperoni-induced heartburn, so watching what you eat can make a difference.

Other steps you can take will ease your heartburn.

- Eat small meals or healthy snacks throughout the day instead of three big meals.

- Eat slowly and chew thoroughly.

- Don't bend over at your waist. Bend at your knees instead (also a good way to preserve your back).

- Elevate your head slightly when you sleep at night.

- Chew gum after meals. (But stay away from aspartame sweetener and peppermint or spearmint flavors, all of which can aggravate the problem.)

Between food aversions carried over from the first trimester and heartburn, your daily menu choices may dwindle. Be creative when finding other foods to help you maintain a healthy diet.

Chafing

You may still squeeze into your favorite shorts and running bra, but they don't fit like they did 2 months ago. Seams can rub against tender areas—most often your underarms, bra region, and inner thighs. Sometimes you won't even realize you've been chafed until the shower water stings you.

This might be a good time to invest in a new pair of shorts, bra, or other piece of clothing that will alleviate the irritation. Choose fabrics that wick away sweat efficiently. Bras with nylon linings are gentlest on skin. If chafing continues:

- Rub petroleum jelly or runners' lubricant on the tender areas before you run. (Chap Stick works in a pinch, and you can easily carry it in your pocket while you run.)

- Tuck a scrap of moleskin between the tender skin and your clothing.

- Turn your running bra, shorts, tights, or shirt inside out to keep seams away from your skin.

- After your shower, rub an antibiotic ointment like Neosporin on the chafed skin and cover it loosely with sterile gauze to promote healing.

YOUR CONCERNS

Dizziness

Remember back in the first trimester when you felt lightheaded half the time? The problem most likely went away after your blood volume caught up with your expanding circulatory system. As your pregnancy progresses, the growing baby may put extra pressure on your blood vessels, causing the dizziness to come back. You may notice it especially when you rise from a seated or prone position too quickly.

If you feel dizzy while running, try not to stop suddenly, which can cause blood to pool in your veins and intensify your dizziness. "Slow down and try to find a place to hold yourself up, like a wall," says Dr. Kulpa. Lying down on your left side is the best way to cope with prenatal dizziness—but rarely practical when you're out on a run. Try sitting down with your head between your knees until the dizziness recedes. You can attempt to run again if the feeling disappears completely. Otherwise, walk home or call for a ride.

Sometimes low blood sugar causes dizziness. Avoid this problem by eating balanced meals throughout the day, along with a small snack 1 hour before

> ## Stand Up to Muscle Strain
>
> Dizziness isn't the only hazard of standing up too quickly. If you stand up wrong, you may strain muscles or ligaments. "Use your arms and legs instead of your back," says Patty Kulpa, M.D., a sports gynecologist in Gig Harbor, Washington. Practice getting out of bed the proper way: Lie on your side and push yourself up with your hands while letting your legs swing down to the floor like a pendulum. As your belly grows, the "pendulum" method of rising becomes increasingly important.

your workout. See chapter 4 for foods that will nourish your exercise and your baby.

Many runners choose carbohydrates for their preworkout snack. Mix in some protein to stave off hunger and dizziness. Some examples: a broiled cheese sandwich (with a single slice of cheese so that you don't overdo your prerun fat intake); cereal, milk, and berries; or a small turkey sandwich. Experiment to find out what works best for your pregnant running body.

You can also bring some easy-to-carry treats with you for emergencies. Sports gels, granola bars, dried fruit, and the like will help you perk up if your energy levels plummet on the trail. Don't forget to eat after your workout to keep your body well-stocked for tomorrow's run.

Safety

As a pregnant runner, you stand out from the crowd, and that means you can be a target of violence. It's always a good idea before you leave to tell someone your running route and the estimated length of time you'll be gone. Also, carry identification (with your name, phone number, and blood type).

All runners should have a game plan for what they'll do if approached, says Paul Henry Danylewich, director of White Tiger Street Defense in Montreal, Quebec, and author of the book *Fearless: The Complete Personal Safety Guide for Women*. In other words, come up with and practice standard reactions for potential situations. For example, if a person stops his car and rolls down the window, you will not walk closer. "Never let a potential threat get closer than 3 to 5 feet of you," Danylewich says. Another example: You will run away from an attacker rather than trying to fight.

Of course, you won't need to use these plans if you never have a problem in the first place. Stay safe by not running in unpopulated or unfamiliar areas. Know which stores are open and which houses you

Get Along, Little Doggie

Loose dogs love runners. With few exceptions, an unconfined dog must come and check you out. It is a biological imperative. The problem is that you probably don't want company on your run, especially the kind of company that could bite. So what do you do if you run by a dog and it perks its head up? "Immediately stop running," says Stephanie Shain, director of outreach for companion dogs and a dog-bite expert with the Humane Society of the United States in Washington, D.C. "Continue walking slowly." If the dog starts to chase, stand still and don't make eye contact. "We think of eye contact as a sign of respect, but to a dog it's a challenge," Shain says. Stand quietly and let the dog sniff you. Don't give in to your urge to yell or run away, since this will arouse its interest even more.

It's often hard to tell if a dog is about to attack: It may growl or simply stand alert with its ears and tail up, or it may give no indication at all. Try to stay on your feet during an attack and protect your head and belly. "If you get knocked down, curl into a ball, tuck your head in, protect your face and put your fists over your ears," Shain says.

Seek medical help after an attack, and make sure your obstetrician knows what has happened. "Don't forget to call your local animal control, humane society, or local law enforcement," Shain says. "You'll want to do that as soon as possible, especially if the dog is running at large."

could run to for help. If you must run after dark, do so only in well-lit areas. And vary your routine—don't run the same route at the same time every day.

It's good to make a habit of looking people in the eye as you run by them. This projects an air of confidence, making you a less obvious target, and lets would-be attackers know you could identify them. If you come upon a group of men, run around them or cross the street. And ignore verbal harassment—you don't want to call any more attention to yourself. Other strategies include:

- Run with a friend or your dog.

(continued on page 140)

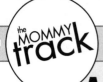

A SPEEDSTER SLOWS DOWN
FOR MOTHERHOOD

Name: Linda Gill

Birth date: June 1958

Residence: San Anselmo, California

Occupation: Coach to individual high school runners

Children: Four daughters, born 1986, 1987, 1993, 1996

FROM RACER TO RUNNER

Once upon a time, Linda Gill was a California high school track star, winning the state mile her senior year and earning a scholarship to the University of California, Los Angeles. She remained a competitive middle-distance runner even after her first two children were born. Clearly, she wasn't about to let a simple pregnancy (or four) keep her from the sport she loved.

So she played it safe. During her pregnancy runs, Linda made sure to keep her heart rate under 130, following the advice of her doctor. She didn't want to push herself too hard. "If you're in good shape, you can push yourself more than you should, without realizing it," she says. "That was always my fear." During every pregnancy but the second, she ran with ease, getting out four or five times a week and even completing her regular Sunday 11-miler into the eighth month. Surprisingly, her last pregnancy was the easiest. The day before she delivered, she ran 4 miles and noted in her journal, "I can't believe how nothing hurts."

When she wanted to do speedwork, she shifted her track workout to the stationary bike. Stationary cycling kept her heart rate in the prescribed range and gave her burgeoning body a break from pounding on pavement. It also allowed her to exercise through her second pregnancy, when pain seared her lower abdomen and forced her to stop running. "The second one was only 20 months younger than my first," she says. "I think my abdominal area hadn't gotten strong again."

Even when she felt good, she resisted the temptation to race while pregnant because she worried about hurting the baby. Instead, she saved races for in between pregnancies. "My goal was to have a kid, try to get into shape again, have a kid, try to get into shape again," she laughs.

FROM RUNNER TO WALKER

Linda didn't make the same mistakes a lot of other enthusiastic runners make postdelivery. For starters, C-section deliveries of all her children required that she slowly ease back into running. She walked until 6 weeks postpartum, then transitioned to short, slow jogs.

FROM MOTHER TO DAUGHTERS

The running bug recently bit Linda's oldest daughter, who joined the high school cross-country team upon starting her junior year. "She fought it as long as she could," Linda says. "Now she's in the top five in the county." The contagion spread through the family. Linda's second and third daughters now run track. "I attend a lot of meets," she says. She squeezes in her own runs between her kids' sporting events and her coaching duties. "I make running a priority. You can always find time to do something you think is important."

LINDA'S TIPS

Run your own pregnancy. Don't compare yourself to anyone else. Every pregnancy is different. See how you're feeling before you decide how much running you'll do.

Get back slowly. After the baby is born and you start feeling better, you will probably forget that not everything inside your body is where it's supposed to be. Give your body time to get back to normal before you resume running.

Choose running partners wisely. When you run with people who don't have kids, they won't understand how hard it is for you to get out there. And they probably won't cut you any slack.

- Stay alert. That means leaving your headphones at home and paying attention to people around you.

- Run at a pace that won't leave you out of breath if you're faced with a confrontation.

- Carry a cell phone and telephone numbers to summon help.

- Run in the opposite direction of traffic so that you can see the cars passing you.

- Trust your intuition about a person or an area.

- Practice memorizing license tags or identifying characteristics of strangers.

- Take a self-defense class from a qualified instructor.

If you do end up in a situation where you feel threatened, screaming is the most effective distress signal. People notice it more than they do a whistle or portable alarm, and you can do it without wasting precious seconds fumbling around in your pocket. "Portable alarms can break," Danylewich says. "And we've seen cases in which the pepper spray has been used against someone or the spray has blown back into the person's face." Finally, "never go anywhere with an aggressor, even if he displays a weapon," Danylewich says. "Any place he takes you is sure to be far more isolated."

Keeping Up with Running Partners

Running with a buddy or group is a safe choice, since the likelihood of being attacked decreases when you're with others. And it's fun to have people with whom to talk and share encouragement. The only problem when you're pregnant is keeping up with them. Right now, you need to listen to your body and respect the pace it's setting for you. When it compels you to slow down, you need to obey, even if that means holding up the group or waving them ahead.

It might help to run with fellow pregnant runners who've slowed their pace just like you. Ask your obstetrician for names of other pregnant runners, post a notice in her waiting room, ask around at your health club, or ask your local running club for names. "The social benefit, the confidence, and the empowerment you can derive from those other runners is exceptional," says Frank Webbe, Ph.D., professor of psychology at Florida Institute of Technology in Melbourne and president of a group called the Running Psychologists.

Restraining Your Competitive Nature

Many runners have a favorite road race they run each year. You're probably no different. Your pregnancy doesn't have to stop you, but if you're a competitive runner, you'll need to tone down your efforts. "Among top-level competitors in the running community, there's an undercurrent of who can run the farthest into their pregnancy and do the most," says triathlete Keller. "It's what I'd call bragging rights." While it's great for your fitness level, it's not so great for your pregnancy.

You don't have to be an elite runner to feel competitive. Just participating in your local 5-K can make you want to pour on the heat. It's disappointing to be farther back in the pack than you're used to. But remember that pride matters very little in the grand scheme of things; the way you treat your pregnant body (and the baby inside it) matters a great deal.

To run a race without actually competing, plan ahead, says Judy Van Raalte, Ph.D., a runner, mother of two, and professor of psychology at Springfield College in Massachusetts. Try to find a slower runner or a new runner who needs encouragement and run with her. "Or volunteer and hand out juice instead," says Dr. Van Raalte. "That way you can still be part of the race, and you can run it again safely next year."

CHAPTER 10

THE SIXTH MONTH

RUNNING STRONG

IT'S A GOOD THING speed doesn't count right now. If you charted your running efforts on a graph these days, the line representing your running times would curve upward. Last week it took you 9 minutes to run to the neighborhood park, this week 10, and so on. You never imagined you'd get so slow—and you're not even in the third trimester yet.

PREGNANCY STEPBY**STEP**

Month 6: You have become a neighborhood institution. Every runner, walker, and cyclist on your route knows you by sight. Inside the womb, your baby opens her eyes.

Strength does count, and as a pregnant runner, you are among the very strongest of athletes, physically and mentally. "Each time you go out, you demonstrate what you can do," says Frank Webbe, Ph.D., professor of psychology at Florida Institute of Technology in Melbourne and president of a group called the Running Psychologists. "Realizing that you are staying in shape should make you feel good about your body."

FEELINGS AND SENSATIONS

The Pelvic Floor Dance

Before midpregnancy, you may have been puzzled by the term *pelvic floor*. It's a safe bet that you've got it figured out now. The baby grows and puts pressure on the muscles between your legs; we veterans call it the Pelvic Floor Dance. Pelvic floor muscles create a sling or hammock reaching from your pubic bone to your tailbone. Unlike other parts of your pelvis, which are supported by bone, this area is flexible and springy.

Pregnancy and childbirth stretch and subsequently weaken these muscles—specifically the pubococcygeal (PC) muscles. Strengthening them can help you in two ways. First, strong pelvic floor muscles may help decrease the injuries you sustain during childbirth and help you recover more quickly postpartum. "As with strengthening any muscle in your body, you're actually creating tissue that's more elastic and more supple and will slide out of the way more easily during delivery," says Joy Backstrum, a physical therapist in Anchorage, Alaska. Second, strong pelvic floor muscles help prevent stress incontinence (accidentally urinating when you run, sneeze, cough, or laugh) after your baby is born.

Find your PC muscles by stopping and then starting your urine flow. Once you're sure of their location, you can work on your "form." Concentrate your efforts on the middle section of your vagina rather than the opening, and contract your pelvic floor muscles inward and upward. After your initial try, perform Kegel exercises when you aren't urinating, since continuing to interrupt your urine flow can inhibit your ability to void easily.

Begin with a routine of 5-second holds with 10-second rests in between, and work your way up to 10-second holds with 10- to 20-second rests in between. Spend a minimum of 5 minutes on Kegels three to four times a week.

To get even more benefit from Kegels, consider the muscles that make up the pelvic floor. You've likely read about fast-twitch and slow-twitch muscle fibers. In your legs, the fast-twitch muscle fibers help power short, hard bursts of energy, while the slow-twitch fibers come into play for endurance activities. These muscles also structure your pelvic floor—slow-twitch fibers in the deepest layers of muscle and fast-twitch in the more superficial layers. To strengthen both types of muscle fibers, Backstrum offers these suggestions: "Do strongholds (Kegels at maximum effort) and quick-flicks (contracting for 2 seconds, relaxing for 4)." Backstrum recommends that patients break up their Kegel routines into two or three smaller sessions throughout the day and practice them in different positions, as described on the previous page.

Here are some tips on getting the most from Kegels.

- If you find Kegels difficult, start by repeating your 5-second holds just 5 times. Then move on to 8- to 10-second holds, repeating 10 times, before working up to a full 5 minutes.

- Pull your pelvic floor muscles inward and upward, similar to how the vagina grips the penis during intercourse.

- Concentrate on pulling inward and upward from midway up your vagina instead of from the opening.

- Resist the urge to bear down. Try to imagine holding something inside yourself rather than pushing it out.

- Try not to involve the buttocks or thigh muscles. "It is okay to contract your abdominal muscles," says Backstrum. "They are neurologically connected to the pelvic floor, and you can't isolate them."

- Practice the exercises in different positions, such as lying on your back (but not after the fourth month), side, and stomach; on your hands and knees; standing; and sitting. This will help you effectively use the pelvic floor muscles in a variety of situations.

- To evaluate whether you're doing Kegels correctly, place a finger in your vagina up to the second knuckle, Backstrum says. "If you press back and to the side, that is actually the bulk of the muscle tissue. Do what you think is a Kegel and if you feel thickening of the tissue or the muscle contraction underneath your fingertip, you're probably doing it correctly."

Brain Fog

One of the more disturbing side effects of pregnancy is also the most mysterious. How can you go from sharp, rational go-getter to distracted, less-than-rational pregnant woman in the space of just a few months? How can such a small baby overtake your body and claim your brain, too?

Highs and Lows of Running during Pregnancy

Highs

- Knowing you'll never again have to work so hard to run so slowly
- Sleep
- Endorphin buzz (the only kind you're still allowed)
- Forgetting you're pregnant
- High-fives from other runners
- Picturing the hot mama you'll be when it's all over

Lows

- Your new "outie" poking through your running shorts
- Curious stares from perfect strangers
- Shared opinions from perfect strangers
- Your pancake-shaped bladder
- The kielbasa syndrome (or squeezing into your running shorts)
- Gas

A few theories compete for our feeble attention. One is that a pregnant woman's brain shrinks during the third trimester, presumably as a result of the hormones circulating through it. Another theory is that we have too much to think about, with planning for the baby's arrival, imagining being his mom, working, exercising, and so forth. A third theory suggests that we're busy communing with the baby, even though we might not realize it.

A handful of studies during the past 10 years has linked vigorous exercise with improved mental acuity. Although there is no direct link between exercise and *prenatal* mental acuity, many women claim it helps. "I felt like I had lost my mind during pregnancy," says Judy Van Raalte, Ph.D., a runner, mother of two, and professor of psychology at Springfield College in Massachusetts. "Running helped because it gave me time to think."

If you find yourself spacing out regularly, it may mean you need some rest. Take a day off from your workouts and see if you feel lucid again. If not, try running in safe places like around the neighborhood track or municipal golf course. Remember that inattention can get you into trouble. Force yourself to be alert and notice who and what is around you. Ask your doctor to check or recheck you for anemia at your next visit. Iron deficiency makes you sluggish and could contribute to your brain fog.

Boredom

Every runner gets bored now and then—even the most dedicated. It's easy to fall into a rut and let running become ho-hum. The pressures of pregnancy—both psychological and physical—don't help. Family members may openly worry about you and the baby when you run, despite all the information you've given them. On top of that, you now feel the baby's weight with every stride. It's easy to wonder, "Why do I bother?"

If you're exceptionally uncomfortable, now might be a good time to switch to some other form of exercise that doesn't increase your

(continued on page 150)

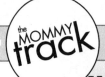

NO CHALLENGE TOO GREAT

Name: Lisa Keller

Birth date: January 1964

Residence: Anchorage

Occupation: Running coach for adults and high school kids

Children: Two, born 1997 and 2000

A CHANGE OF PERSPECTIVE

Lisa Keller is always itching for a challenge. In 1984, when she was a college student and runner, Lisa competed in her first triathlon and fell in love with the sport. A committed triathlete ever since, she has been both race director and winner of the Alaska Women's Gold Nugget Triathlon, the oldest all-women's triathlon in the United States.

But some challenges she could do without. In 2002, Lisa was diagnosed with breast cancer. Facing this disease made all her other accomplishments seem easy. Triathlons? Piece of cake. Pregnancy? A breeze. Staying fit during pregnancy? No problem.

When Lisa became pregnant for the first time in 1997, she didn't think twice about continuing to run. "I've been a runner all my life, so it wasn't even a conscious choice," she says. She ran for 30 to 45 minutes about four times a week, folding in some biking and swimming. She exercised conservatively, while keeping her mind on racing. "A lot of my motivation is gone if I'm not racing," she says. "I was trying to be in the best shape possible so, after the pregnancy was over, I could work toward competing again."

After recovering from the birth of her first daughter in December 1997, Lisa began training for the May 1998 Gold Nugget Triathlon (in which she placed third). By the next year, she was in top condition and won the same event. Just 3 months after that, she won an Olympic-distance triathlon in Washington state called the Titanium Man. That very night, she conceived her second daughter.

Lisa ran most of the way through her second pregnancy, too, but was sidelined during the sixth month by a case of shingles. Undeterred, Lisa resumed cycling as soon as she could stand to wear a sports bra again.

RACING ON HER MIND

After delivery, Lisa followed her doctor's recommendation to wait until she stopped bleeding to run again. "Of course, in both my pregnancies that was a full 6 weeks," she says. She was able to go for walks at 2 weeks, and at the 6-week marks, she started a walk-run program. "After the first pregnancy, it was February; it was cold and it was snowing," says Lisa. "I felt sloppy—my stomach was bouncing up and down, my chest was bouncing up and down. But I was so excited to be out there."

After her breast cancer diagnosis, Lisa attacked the disease with the same aggressiveness she employs for racing. Only this time, she swapped her strenuous program of swimming, biking, and running for a new (and much more grueling) schedule of surgery, chemotherapy, and radiation. At the time she shared her story for this book, Lisa was still undergoing treatment.

Her desire to compete gets her through the treatments, just as it motivated her during her pregnancies. "I keep thinking, 'I'm going to win the survivor division in the Alaska Run for Women,'" she says. "'And then I'll go to the Lower 48 and run some Susan Komen Races for the Cure.'"

LISA'S TIPS

Remember the intrinsic benefits of exercise. Running gives you power, makes you feel good about yourself, and gives you a sense of control.

Carve out time for exercise. After your baby is born, your exercise time becomes your alone time. And it may be the only time you get!

Set a goal. If you like to race, plan to enter a women's race 4 to 6 months after your baby is born. That gives you a goal for getting back into competition.

discomfort. If you've been cross-training once or twice a week already, you may already be familiar with something that works. If not, figure out what else you like to do and work into it slowly.

If you're in a run-of-the-mill slump, remember that you're an athlete—pregnant or not. Athletes get out the door every day. Your pregnancy merely adds a new challenge—and isn't challenge what being an athlete is all about? Picture yourself a year from now. What you do today contributes to how you'll perform then.

Here are some more ways to break through the doldrums.

Set goals. Long-range goals—a 5-K 4 months after delivery or even a marathon 10 months after you give birth—give you something to think of beyond your current state of misery, even if you change them later.

Readjust short-term goals. "First trimester I ran my usual mileage, but then each of the following trimesters, I cut my running back by a third," says Dr. Van Raalte. "I reduced my expectations, and since I was meeting my goals, I wasn't disappointed."

Use your head. Every athlete knows that running is more than bodywork. It involves mental and spiritual components as well. Pregnancy gives you the space to focus on these aspects of the sport. New scenery stimulates your mind and senses, so find some different routes. If you can't think of another place to run, ask your friends. Or run your old route in reverse. You'll notice things you didn't spot going the other way. Concentrate on what you're seeing, smelling, hearing, and feeling, and go home and jot them in your running journal.

Read your running journal. It will remind you of what you've accomplished thus far. You're still running nearly two-thirds of the way through your pregnancy. That makes you an inspiration to other people. Why not to yourself?

Create theme runs. Study people's holiday decorations. Count how many fire hydrants you pass. Award "prizes" for the most original landscaping. Do anything to distract yourself from your own footfalls.

Plan rewards for your effort. A pedicure, a massage, or an ice cream cone go a long way toward making your effort seem worthwhile. And don't forget that running can be its own reward. "The energy I got from it was incredible," says Shannon Avery, a Puerto Rico–based runner and mother of two. "I had more energy afterward if I just moved myself out the door when I didn't want to go."

Stop clocking your times. Occasionally ignorance really is bliss, especially if your pregnancy-induced slowdown disheartens you.

Find a running buddy. Another pregnant runner will likely run at your pace and understand everything you're experiencing. Or try going out with a slower runner, since your paces may be more evenly matched. If you were a slow runner to begin with, find a brand-new runner who needs coaching.

Volunteer at a road race. Seeing hundreds of other runners, feeling the excitement of the race, and doing something nice for others will recharge your batteries.

When all else fails, take a few days off. Sometimes the itch to run returns all on its own.

YOUR CONCERNS

Edema

Though it sounds like something requiring quarantine, it's really the "normal" swelling of your feet and ankles during pregnancy. With the increase in fluid circulating through your body, it's not surprising that some of it collects in your lower extremities. Staying hydrated, avoiding excessive amounts of salt, and keeping your feet elevated when possible can help.

Dr. Kulpa advises patients with edema not to run. Swollen tissue is more susceptible to injury, she says. "Also, runners won't have a good sense of the impact on their feet." Shoes can begin to fit poorly, which can cause soft-tissue problems like blisters and black toenails. If your feet, ankles, or lower legs begin to swell, stop running and ask your doctor what type of cross-training you can do safely.

If your face or hands become puffy, stop all exercise and call your doctor to make sure you aren't suffering from preeclampsia (also known as *toxemia* or *hypertension*). Untreated, preeclampsia can cause numerous problems and affect the growth of the placenta, your baby's lifeline. If it progresses to eclampsia, both of your lives will be in danger.

Gestational Diabetes

Between weeks 24 and 28, your doctor will schedule your glucose tolerance test. For most women, this test rules out the possibility of gestational diabetes. Others may need a more extensive follow-up test. These results will show whether you've developed gestational diabetes, a condition in which your body's production of insulin—the hormone that regulates glucose—cannot keep up with the amount of glucose in your blood.

During the third trimester, your body will naturally develop a resistance to insulin. This resistance ensures that the baby will have an adequate supply of glucose, but it also can cause a surplus of glucose in your bloodstream. In a normal pregnancy, your body will create more insulin to deal with the excess glucose. If you have gestational diabetes, you will not be able to produce enough insulin or your body won't be able to use the insulin it does make.

So where does your running fit in? In addition to helping prevent gestational diabetes in the first place, exercise helps fight your body's resistance to insulin. That means that runners with gestational diabetes are often told by their doctors to keep running or cross-training until the end, unless the diabetes has created additional complications (such as high blood pressure or blood vessel damage).

If you're one of the 3 to 5 percent of pregnant women who develop gestational diabetes, follow your doctor's orders to the letter. If she doesn't say anything about your running, remind her that you run, and make sure it's safe to continue. In some cases you'll need to coordinate your workouts with dietary and medication schedules. When given a choice, schedule your test no later than the 24th or 25th week. If it turns out you have gestational diabetes, you'll want to start managing it as soon as possible.

PART 4:
THE THIRD TRIMESTER

CHAPTER 11

THE SEVENTH MONTH

REMODELING YOUR RUNNING PROGRAM

WHEN I REACHED THE 20-MILE MARK in my first marathon, a man on the sidelines yelled, "Congratulations! You're halfway there." I knew instinctively what he meant: The hardest part, the real test of my strength, lay ahead in those last 6.2 miles. And he was right.

> **PREGNANCY**
> **STEP**BY**STEP**
>
> Month 7: You drink a liter of water during your 3-miler. Your baby hiccups.

So goes it with the last trimester of pregnancy. You've undoubtedly been anticipating this time, wondering if it will be as hard as everyone says, questioning if you will still run when your belly feels more like a watermelon than a cantaloupe. Running typically becomes less and less enjoyable as the weeks pass, which is especially disappointing if you sailed through the second trimester. Some of the things you take for granted about your body will change yet again, and you will need to make adjustments.

That said, running is still worth pursuing. Those benefits you've enjoyed all along—better sleep, improved digestion, more consistent moods—are especially important now that pregnancy-related discomforts are at their worst. You may feel more self-conscious in your big running shorts, but you should also feel a sense of pride.

FEELINGS AND SENSATIONS

Unmotivated

The quality of your runs during the seventh month can vary. Some days you'll feel pretty good, some days not so good, and some days your running will go from good to bad every few minutes. While you used to shoot out the door without a second thought, now you have second, third, and fourth thoughts all related to the sentiment "Why should I bother when my runs feel so bad?"

It's hard not to become disappointed in yourself. Your body doesn't react to anything the way it once did—not food, not sleep, and certainly not running. You'll be lucky if your run today felt better than it did yesterday. The mere fact that you're still running is an accomplishment. Try to remember that you're not setting any records right now; you're simply providing continuity between the running you did before you got pregnant and what you plan to do after your baby is born.

Most of all, don't feel guilty if you stop running now or if you stopped a month ago. Sometimes a sixth sense—or plain old common sense—tells you it's quitting time. It's just not worth the discomfort anymore. "The last few weeks of pregnancy, I didn't do much of any kind of exercise," says Lisa Keller, an Anchorage, Alaska, triathlete and mother of two. "I thought, 'At this point, who cares?'"

Make your decision with confidence and pat yourself on the back for running this far into your pregnancy. "There is evidence that a woman will not lose nearly the amount of fitness she thinks she will,"

Hitting the Wall

If you've ever hit the wall in a marathon, you know what it's like to have the road stretch out in front of you like taffy, extending the finish line to some distant, unknowable place. The final weeks of your pregnancy are like that, too, especially since you really *can't* see the finish line. Your pregnancy begins to feel like a permanent condition.

Running does two things to help the way you perceive time. First, it improves the way your body feels—and the better you feel, the faster time seems to pass. Second, it helps you achieve a personal goal, yours alone amid the flurry of projects at home and at work. Review your running journal for a tangible reminder of your efforts. Seeing on paper all the months you've put behind you can reinforce visually that you truly are closer to the finish.

says James Pivarnik, Ph.D., professor of kinesiology and osteopathic surgical specialties and director of the Human Energy Research Laboratory at Michigan State University in East Lansing. "She doesn't have to be a maniac about training up until she delivers."

Sleep Deprived

Starting in the seventh month, sleep may begin to escape you more often than it has up till now. When you lie down at night, it's easier to notice all the room your baby takes up and how much he wiggles. You may have to visit the bathroom more frequently and pop an antacid while you're there, because heartburn is worst at night. And of course you'll worry, as all expectant mothers do, about what is ahead.

As a runner, you're probably aware that running can make you sleep better if you time it right. This is especially important to remember now. Exercise elevates your body temperature slightly, which makes you more alert. Later, as your temperature returns to normal, you'll start to feel sleepy. When you run 3 to 4 hours before bed, you give your body time to complete this cycle.

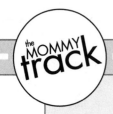

the MOMMY track

LIFE GOES ON

Name: Lauri Brockmiller

Birth date: October 1974

Home: Royal Oak, Michigan

Occupation: Exercise physiologist and personal trainer

Children: One on the way

INSPIRED BY OTHERS

Exercise is Lauri Brockmiller's life. She's not only a runner, triathlete, and adventure racer but also a personal trainer. That's why when she became pregnant she didn't think twice about continuing her running. After all, she's worked with pregnant athletes and observed the benefits they gained from prenatal exercise. "They inspired me to think I could do it, too," she says.

Upon learning she was pregnant, Lauri kept running but slowed her pace from an 8:30 to about a 9:40 mile in the first trimester, and finally to a 10-minute mile in the second trimester. And she cut her first trimester 4-milers back to 3 by the second trimester.

Lauri felt slightly nauseated and more than slightly tired during her first trimester. The fatigue reared its head again at different times throughout the pregnancy, and she dealt with each episode individually. Sometimes she allowed herself to take the day off; other times she pushed herself through the workout. "And then I always felt better," she says.

It was under the worst kind of duress that she quit running. "It got to the point where I was just pounding my bladder," she says. Undaunted, she switched to the elliptical trainer and also started a walking regimen. Lauri who was 8 months pregnant when interviewed, finds that the elliptical trainer causes the least discomfort to her bladder but provides a less intense workout than running. "I work out longer on it," she says, "45 to 60 minutes, sometimes more."

BALANCING STRENGTH AND STAMINA

Lauri continues to strength train throughout the pregnancy. She lifts weights three times a week and does light abdominal exercises regularly. "It doesn't really feel like I'm working my abs. I'm just trying to keep my brain in touch with those muscle groups," she says.

Lauri counsels pregnant athletes not to become discouraged when they feel weaker during pregnancy. "The reason your strength goes down so much is you really can't use your core," she says. "You can only use your body parts." The strength comes back within a few weeks or months postpartum, once mothers can rely on their abdominals again.

NEXT STEPS

Lauri hopes to resume running 2 to 4 weeks postpartum. "I know this isn't textbook," she says. "So if it takes me 2 months, fine. If it takes me 1 week, that's great." She hopes to run some favorite 5-Ks and 10-Ks within a couple of months and maybe complete an 8- to 10-mile run 4 to 5 months down the line.

Three of Lauri's proudest accomplishments are a half Ironman Triathlon, a full marathon, and a multisport adventure race in which she and her team came in third in an all-women's division. If all goes well, she will join the adventure race circuit again about a year after she has her baby.

LAURI'S TIPS

Decipher your body's signals. Listen to your body—but don't be a wimp, either. You need to learn how to tell the difference between when your body is a little sluggish and when you should be lying down.

Reset your priorities. Don't worry about decreases in your running speed. Concentrate on putting in the minutes, and that will help when you're done.

Be a know-it-all. Educate yourself about exercise and pregnancy so when someone asks you, "Should you be doing that?" you can say, "Yes, because [insert great reason here] . . . "

YOUR CONCERNS

Cosmetic Changes

If you're like most pregnant women, you've probably realized that everything changes when you're pregnant. Your appetite, your emotions, and your running pace each undergo such drastic transformation that you may no longer recognize yourself. So you shouldn't be surprised when, at about this time, your skin decides to get into the act, becoming a canvas for a host of unwanted designs.

Stretch marks: You can't do much about these red or pink striations on your abdomen, breasts, hips, or inner thighs. You'll get stretch marks if you're predisposed to them, and they'll be worse if you gain excessive amounts of weight. Stretch marks will fade somewhat after pregnancy. Running won't make much of a difference except to help keep your weight gain in the normal range.

Linea nigra and other skin discolorations: The linea nigra (also known as the ripe stripe) gives your belly that double-hemisphere look. Before pregnancy, it was invisible and called the *linea alba*, or white line. Nowadays it's brown or black and very visible, especially if you have dark skin. The linea nigra will fade after pregnancy, but you may always retain a pale version of it in the area under your belly button.

You may also develop dark patches (if you have light skin) or light patches (if you have dark skin) on your face and in areas of high friction, such as your inner thighs. The sun's rays can make the patches look worse, so wear sunscreen on your face if you notice discoloration. The problem should disappear after pregnancy.

Varicose and spider veins: Varicose veins result from an increase in blood pressure in the legs, where weakened valves allow blood to pool in the veins. For women who are predisposed, veins will start to bulge right along with the belly. This is bad news for runners, who spend more time than most people in shorts and who often take pride in the appearance of their legs. The good news is that running

Altered States

Your body is a wonder as it changes to accommodate the growing baby. Here's what you might experience this month.

- Noticeable separation in your abdominal muscles (called *diastasis recti*)
- Widening and broadening of the belly
- Widening of your rib cage
- Less room between your belly and breasts, which can transform your running bra into a chafing mechanism
- Protruding belly button
- Slumped posture: hunched shoulders, arched lower back, distended neck (to correct this, stand up straighter by tucking your tailbone under, rotating your breastbone up and back a few degrees, and tucking in your chin slightly)
- Knock-kneed stance (if you are standing on the insides of your arches, roll your feet until you feel your weight on the middle portion, and unlock your knees)

If you have a roomy abdominal cavity, you may not experience all of these changes. Your baby load will be spread more evenly throughout your pelvis rather than tugging on the forward section.

can help you avoid varicose veins because it improves circulation. However, if your varicose veins feel tender or outright painful, switch to lower-impact exercise to avoid traumatizing them further. With luck your problem will get better or disappear soon after you've had the baby.

Spider veins may appear on your thighs or face sometime within the third trimester. These enlarged superficial blood vessels are as ugly as they sound and can sometimes be painful, although they should not keep you from running. Some spider veins will fade or disappear after pregnancy and breastfeeding are behind you, and the more persistent ones can be removed surgically. But wait until after you're finished having children: Another pregnancy could cause the veins to reappear somewhere else on your legs.

You can take a few measures to keep varicose and spider veins from getting worse.

- Don't stand for long periods of time.

- Keep a stool under your desk on which to rest your feet and take pressure off your legs.

- Move your legs and feet around during long stretches of sitting.

- Get up and walk around every 30 to 45 minutes when possible.

- Don't sit with your legs crossed.

- Eat high-fiber foods to avoid constipation, which can contribute to varicose veins, especially in the groin area.

- Wear compression-style running shorts for running only; don't spend extra time in them because constricting your lower torso can make varicose veins worse.

- Ask your doctor about support pantyhose if you think you can tolerate them. Pull them on before getting out of bed in the morning.

- Avoid excessive weight gain.

Anticipation of Childbirth

Here's a paradox unique to expectant mothers: You look forward to your last day of pregnancy with equal parts of impatience and terror. You want the discomfort to end, but the only way through it is pain—serious pain.

Because the seventh month marks the beginning of the end, you may begin to feel the fear now. Maybe you dream about childbirth. Maybe you've read too many books. Maybe your friends with kids have begun to regale you with their own childbirth stories in the name of providing helpful advice. Whatever the case, running can alleviate your fears. Studies have shown that for pregnant women who exercise, labor is shorter and involves fewer complications. Athletes who have endured labor say that their training gave them a mental edge during childbirth.

When I was pregnant for the first time and working out on a stair-climbing machine, I "trained" for contractions. Five or six times during each workout, I notched up the level of difficulty for 1 minute so that I could concentrate on the length of a contraction. (Contractions are 60 to 90 seconds long during the last, most painful phase of labor.) I don't know if it made a whit of difference during the real thing, but it gave me purpose along the way.

The best thing you can do to calm your fears is to choose a childbirth education class if you haven't already. Study the classes available in your area. Many start 7 or 8 weeks before your due date and continue for 6 weeks, although some start much earlier in the pregnancy.

Most childbirth education classes tout the benefits of natural childbirth. Even if you plan to have an epidural or other pain medication, don't ignore what you can gain from these classes. Learning to cope with labor pain is valuable in case there is a gap between your request for pain relief and when you get it. Childbirth education classes often include videotapes of live births; this thought might make you squirm now, but after watching half a dozen of them, you'll feel less queasy about the whole thing.

By selecting a class, you are doing something to make your childbirth experience a little easier. Best of all, you'll meet other expectant mothers with whom you can commiserate.

CHAPTER 12

THE EIGHTH MONTH

FRONT-END LOADED

AROUND MONTH 8, you'll start going to the doctor every 2 weeks instead of every 4, a welcome milestone in your pregnancy. It's hard to imagine looking forward to a gynecologist appointment, but during pregnancy the doctor is your conduit to the baby, and you gain valuable insights at each visit. For example, you'll learn about the baby's presentation: whether she is upside down as she's supposed to be, or right side up, which is called *breech*. Sometime between now and delivery, the baby should turn into the head-down position, and if she doesn't, your doctor may try to rotate her. Some women with breech babies do deliver vaginally, but cesarean section is more common.

> **PREGNANCY STEP**BY**STEP**
>
> Month 8: Your hard-charging runs have become meditation in motion. Some of the fine-tuning of your baby's brain occurs this month.

Besides hanging around upside down and kicking you a lot, what else is your baby doing in there? She is fattening up to about 5 pounds and growing to 18 inches, and her brain is developing rapidly. Her lungs may not be fully mature yet, but she could likely survive outside the womb if you gave birth now. Here's what you're doing, thinking, and feeling.

FEELINGS AND SENSATIONS

Belly Bounce

Big baby translates to big belly, which means you might need extra support when running. Consider investing in a pair of maternity running tights or compression shorts if you haven't already. If that's not enough, add a maternity support belt over your shorts or wear a unitard or swimsuit underneath. Running uphill provides some relief because it reduces belly bounce. Avoid running downhill, or walk the downhill portions of your route, to avoid the extra force on your internal organs.

Generalized Anxiety

As sure as the baby presses on your pelvis, your emotional cares begin to press on you during the eighth or ninth month. You stand at a unique juncture in time, and a slew of questions passes through your mind in rapid succession. Just as you solve one question, another slides in to replace it. Can you stand this pregnancy for another few weeks? Will you be able to tolerate labor and delivery? What if something goes wrong? Are you cut out to be a mother? What if your baby isn't perfect? What if you get postpartum depression?

At night these concerns chip away at your sleep. When this happens, get up and do something to distract yourself. Read a book, watch TV, or get on the treadmill for a walk or jog. If your fears start to bury you during daylight hours, get out and run as soon as possible. "Exercise is a great mood enhancer," says Judy Van Raalte, Ph.D., a runner, mother of two, and professor of psychology at Springfield College in Massachusetts. "It gives you the confidence that you can get through the pregnancy and delivery."

Out of Room

It's true: You're being squeezed out of your own body by a baby. The "little" one begins to occupy every cranny in your abdominal cavity, and you can't breathe deeply, eat a full meal, or drink more than a few sips at a time. Going for a run can help—a little. The endorphins circulating in your blood will make you care less about your bodily eviction, but the jostling may make you feel worse. Try exercising in the pool or taking a deep, cool bath to alleviate some of the baby pressure. When you find a few minutes of privacy, get down on your hands and knees and rest there to allow gravity to pull your baby forward. This will give your own infrastructure a break.

YOUR CONCERNS

Needing a Cesarean

Doctors perform C-sections for a number of reasons, not just breech presentation. In fact, 15 to 20 percent of all deliveries are C-sections, so even if you don't plan to deliver that way, discuss it with your doctor just in case. Many women prefer to deliver vaginally when possible, and especially as a runner, you'll be interested in the difference in recovery times: After an uncomplicated vaginal delivery, your doctor usually will let you return to running 2 to 4 weeks postpartum and sometimes sooner; after a C-section, it's more like 6 to 10 weeks.

C-sections result from a variety of circumstances. They can be scheduled ahead of time, as with a breech baby that cannot be turned; performed on an unscheduled basis, such as when labor is not progressing; and carried out in emergency situations, such as when the baby is in distress. Of course, your doctor is the expert, but if she suggests scheduling a C-section in advance, don't be shy about asking questions to make sure it is necessary. You need to understand all your options, and your doctor needs to know if you consider a C-section a last resort.

Here are some situations in which your doctor may want to schedule a C-section.

- You have pregnancy-induced hypertension (also called *preeclampsia* or *toxemia*) and the rigors of vaginal delivery would endanger you or the baby.

- You have gestational diabetes and your doctor wants to deliver before the baby grows any bigger. Sometimes labor will be induced, but if your cervix is not ready, a C-section may be preferable.

- You have placenta previa, in which the placenta covers or partially covers the "mouth" of the cervix. In this case, labor and delivery could cause you to hemorrhage.

- Your placenta has partially separated from the uterine wall. A very small separation may be treated with bed rest and careful monitoring. (If there is a complete separation, an emergency C-section will be performed.)

- Your baby is overdue by more than a week, your doctor may want to induce your labor or deliver by C-section. Many overdue babies are extra large, and vaginal delivery can be more difficult and complicated, so some doctors prefer C-sections. This may be a gray area, and you should inform your doctor of your preference under these circumstances.

- Your baby is considered *postmature*, that is, overdue by 2 weeks or more, and your doctor determines that the baby's environment in the uterus may be deteriorating.

- If you had a previous C-section that required a vertical incision, you will need to deliver by C-section. Most women who've had a previous C-section with a "bikini" cut can attempt a vaginal delivery in subsequent pregnancies.

You should also discuss reasons your doctor would do an unscheduled or emergency C-section. (These circumstances generally make a C-section nonnegotiable.) Educate yourself now, because when the emergency arises, you won't have time or presence of mind to ask questions. Some common reasons include:

- The doctor detects physical stress in you or the baby before or during labor.

- You have preeclampsia or full-blown eclampsia that has not stabilized with treatment.

- The doctor detects a prolapsed umbilical cord. Occasionally after your water breaks, the cord can slip into the birth canal. Vaginal delivery could cause the baby to compress the cord and cut off her oxygen supply, so a C-section becomes necessary.

- Your labor does not progress despite all efforts and does not respond to contraction-stimulating drugs.

Incontinence

Some women experience—or reexperience—stress incontinence during the third trimester. Wear a pad to catch the leaks. Flat pads with wings will stay in place while you run, although if you don't pull them tightly around your underwear, the wings can chafe your inner thighs. Mention your incontinence to your doctor at the next visit; she may want to confirm you're not leaking amniotic fluid. In the rare instance in which the leaking does not stop after your run, call your doctor right away. If you still suffer incontinence 3 to 6 months postpartum, ask your doctor to refer you to a urogynecologist for testing.

Running at Night

Some people have to run in the dark—it may be the only time a busy schedule permits. Others prefer it; they're night owls who run best in the evening. Despite the research that says exercise before bed will keep us awake, I've always found that an endorphin buzz can be a terrific sleep aid. As long as you take safety precautions, night running won't hurt you. But you do have to work harder at staying hydrated after your run, since you can't drink and sleep at the same time. Build up your fluid intake throughout the day, as well as during and just after your run. Keep a glass of water next to your bed or take a drink in the bathroom each time you get up to pee.

Take It Easy

Your pregnancy pervades every aspect of your life during the third trimester. Your belly interferes with normal day-to-day activities, and you may have even bumped into the doorjamb or knocked something over with your belly. Strangers ask you about your due date; friends who haven't seen you recently raise their eyebrows in surprise. Still, sometimes you forget just how ungainly you've become. Before you make any decisions on the run, ask yourself some of these questions.

- If you're jogging in the road and a driver careens toward you, will you be able to sprint to safety?

- When you hop on or off a curb, can you be sure you'll land where you plan to?

- Do you run on even surfaces?

- Should you stop running while you peel off that extra layer of clothing?

- Do you shuffle your feet? Could you work on lifting your legs a little higher to keep from tripping?

During your warmup, make a promise to yourself to run safely and to remember that some of your small, seemingly mindless choices can have big consequences. Then proceed with caution.

When your hydration levels are low, your bladder can undergo a spasm. Spasms occur when a heavy baby has been sitting on an empty bladder for a while, and the spasms create sharp, continuous pain that will catapult you to the phone to call your doctor. I experienced this one midnight during my first pregnancy and assumed I was going into labor prematurely. The doctor suggested I drink 2 quarts of water over the next 30 minutes and sit in a warm bath. The combination worked. My bladder filled up and resumed its normal position, and the bath helped soothe it.

If you think you're suffering from a bladder spasm, ask your doctor before trying any home remedies, says Ingrid Nygaard, M.D., associate professor of obstetrics and gynecology at the University of Iowa.

"Bladder spasms are not uncommon in pregnancy, but they are hard to differentiate from uterine contractions."

Morning runners have the same hydration issues as night runners, only in reverse. You need to drink water throughout the night so that you can *start* your run well-hydrated. A mid-run bladder spasm would be excruciating.

Learning about Episiotomies

Remember when you learned what an episiotomy was? You probably felt queasy at the prospect of being cut in such a private, sensitive place. (In case you haven't heard the news, an episiotomy is an incision made in your perineum—the area between your vagina and anus—to make the vaginal opening large enough for the baby's head just before birth.)

The theory behind the episiotomy is that it's better to create a straight incision than to allow the haphazard tearing that usually results otherwise. "Sometimes an episiotomy is needed because the baby is in distress and needs to come out fast," says Dr. Nygaard, who has a clinical specialty in urogynecology. "But ultimately it's better for the woman to tear." Here's why: It's true that repairing a complicated ragged tear is harder than repairing a clean episiotomy incision. But a natural tear is less likely to involve the anal sphincter muscle. When that muscle is damaged, the result can be long-term fecal incontinence—releasing stool and gas when you don't intend to. (Read more on fecal incontinence in chapter 14.)

Episiotomies come in two basic forms: median, which goes straight back toward the rectum and puts you at greatest risk for anal sphincter damage, and medio-lateral, which angles away from the rectum and reduces the risk of this kind of damage.

Many women interviewed for this book said that their episiotomy kept them from returning to running as quickly as they would have liked. And at least one study shows that healing from an episiotomy hurts more than healing from spontaneous tearing.

(continued on page 176)

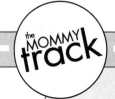

STAYING THE COURSE

Name: Liz Lincoln
Birth date: December 1962
Residence: Lake Forest, Illinois
Occupation: Physical therapist
Children: Three, born 1995, 1997, and 1999

A SACRIFICE NOT WORTH MAKING

One of the driving forces behind Liz Lincoln's pregnant running was her desire to maintain a normal lifestyle. "I gave up my coffee and my wine," she says. "It was nice to still get some good exercise and be able to sweat." Liz continued her regular 25 miles per week throughout the first two trimesters of each pregnancy, cutting back to four 4-mile weekly runs by the end. She strived to keep up a decent pace. "I'd try to get my pace as high as an 8½-minute mile in the last trimester," she says, "even just for a few minutes." (Her nonpregnancy 4-mile pace is 7:45.)

The treadmill, which she used primarily at the end of each pregnancy, softened her footfalls. "The treadmill is just so much bouncier than the pavement," she says. "And the only other places I could run were on the sidewalk or road." Good belly support helped, too. She wore a piece of gear called the Prenatal Cradle that was like a support belt with suspenders that crisscrossed in front and back. "As I got bigger, it kept me more together," she says.

Although she felt a bit self-conscious in the third trimesters, running improved her body image. "Your body goes through some weird things during pregnancy," she says. "But no matter what, you always feel good when you come back from a run." Running helped with her actual body, too. "I think exercise helped keep me from gaining extra weight. I look at pictures, and I didn't look that much different in my face or arms."

MAKING THE SWITCH

Eventually, running gave way to cross-training. Liz ran for 7½ months into each of her first two pregnancies and for 8 months into her third before becoming too uncomfortable. The elliptical trainer turned out to be a good stand-in. She ran without holding on, letting her arms swing. "That made me feel like I was running."

During her third pregnancy, she took a spinning class. Like many runners, she found that it took a while to get into the cycling groove. "My heart rate was getting up so high I bought a monitor to check it out." When she felt winded, she backed off.

Liz didn't follow the standard "wait 6 weeks to run" advice after delivering. Instead, she waited until she stopped bleeding, at about 3 weeks, and stepped back onto the treadmill. The easier landings cushioned her recovering body and helped her ease back into road running. Nowadays, she's back doing the longer races she loves. She ran the Chicago Marathon just before her youngest turned 3. "It was the most unbelievable experience," she says. "I want to do that one again sometime."

LIZ'S TIPS

Make technology your friend. If running becomes physically uncomfortable but you don't feel ready to stop, try some different options. Belly support, better-cushioned shoes, and even a treadmill may help you stay the course.

Learn to love walking. You may never have considered walking to be exercise, but until your postpartum body regains its shape and your internal organs resituate, walking is a good idea.

Strengthen your core. After you deliver and your doctor says it's okay, perform easy abdominal exercises such as pelvic tilts. A strong core will help you with any other exercise.

Maternity-Leave Dreams

By now, your boss and coworkers know that you'll be taking maternity leave and how long you plan to be away. Your childless coworkers may tell you how lucky you are to take time off. They may presume that everything goes back to normal within a couple of weeks and that the rest is just vacation. Maybe that's what you think, too.

Don't kid yourself.

If you've scheduled a 6-week maternity leave, the time will sprint by faster than Marion Jones in the 100-meter dash. You'll be so busy recovering from childbirth, adjusting to sleep deprivation, getting to know your baby, scheduling her feedings, and finalizing child-care details that you'll return to work thinking, "But I never caught up on my sleep. And I'm not back in shape yet." In fact, count yourself lucky if you've even started your walk-run program. For longer maternity leaves—say, 4 to 6 months—you may in fact have time to get into some real running.

Let your doctor know if you prefer she not use the procedure except in an emergency—and insist on a medio-lateral incision if an episiotomy is unavoidable.

Packing Your Hospital Bag

Packing the hospital bag is fun. It's one of those tangible reminders that pregnancy will in fact end. You get to project yourself to the time *after* labor and delivery, when a real baby will fill out (well, sort of) the clothes you so lovingly chose for her. Most pregnancy books detail all the items you'll need for the hospital, so I won't list them here. But I will reinforce one point: Don't plan to wear your pre-pregnancy clothes for your trip home. Pack either maternity clothes or some regular clothes two or three sizes up from your pre-pregnancy size. Starting motherhood with reasonable expectations about your body puts you a step ahead of the wishful thinkers.

Running as a Single Mother

If you're a single mom-to-be, your pregnancy-running experience likely has been no different from anybody else's. Your postpartum running experience will be another story—getting out the door while leaving your baby in good hands becomes a major challenge. Do yourself a favor by figuring out your options now.

Find babysitters. Never think small when it comes to your network; the more people who are part of it, the more chances you will have to run. Have any of your friends offered general assistance? Ask them to commit 1 to 2 hours a week so that you can nap in the beginning and run after you've recovered. Do you have a skill worth trading for child care? My sister-in-law is a hairdresser and gave haircuts and perms to a friend who watched her daughter. Put yourself in a position to have a Plan B and Plan C in case Plan A fails. You can never have too many babysitters. (For more on finding babysitters, see page 208.)

Find a running stroller. If someone is throwing you a baby shower and wants suggestions for gifts, ask if the guests will pitch in for a running stroller or a gift certificate to a store where you can buy one. Use it once your baby has good head control and her pediatrician gives you the thumbs-up.

Take your workout inside. If you can swing it, join a gym with a babysitting service and run on the treadmill. Or see if you can find an affordable treadmill to buy or rent. (Yes, treadmills are mind-numbing, but they're better than not running.)

Revisit your workday. Talk to other parents who run and ask how they squeeze in their workouts. Maybe you can run on your lunch hour or just after work while the baby is still in day care or with a sitter.

Talk to other single mothers. Join a support group for single moms. You will learn invaluable tips and build your network.

CHAPTER 13

THE NINTH MONTH

DESPERATELY SEEKING THE FINISH LINE

THE NINTH-MONTH BELLY is a marvel. Just when you think it can't possibly stretch any farther, it ratchets out another half inch. Maternity clothes that seemed enormous 3 months ago now leave fabric imprints around your navel. To add insult to injury, your legs hit your belly every time you take a stride, and the lack of mobility can be frustrating.

PREGNANCY STEPBYSTEP

Month 9: Your slower pace means you can enjoy the world around you. Take in the sights, the sounds, the smells. Meanwhile, your baby's olfactory system is under construction.

At some point the baby will drop or lighten, which means that he will descend into the pelvic cavity. Lightening produces subtle changes for you. You may notice a downward shift in your baby load and feel like you can take deeper breaths. You may also notice that the baby is squashing your bladder like never before. You could consider lightening good news, a sure sign your body is preparing to give birth. On the other hand, labor could still be another 2 to 4 weeks off, so lightening is no reason to stop running—even if it does slow your run to a shuffle.

During your last few (weekly!) doctor visits, you'll learn about the status of your cervix, namely whether it has dilated (opened) and effaced (thinned out). When this starts happening, count it as evidence that your body is working toward moving the baby out. As with lightening, it doesn't signal an immediate onset of labor. So feel free to keep running as long as your doctor says it's still safe.

If you haven't already, ask your doctor how soon she estimates you can start running again after the baby is born. Find out what complications might make a longer recuperation necessary. If you can remember during all the excitement after the baby is born, ask your doctor again in the hospital. Once you've been through the delivery, she can give you a more accurate estimate. (Remember that you probably won't see her again until your 6-week checkup.)

FEELINGS AND SENSATIONS

A Desire to See It Through

By now you've experienced all the pains of pregnancy running firsthand. If you're still running at this point, now might be a good time for a reality check. If your running causes you discomfort or has begun to feel like a chore, why keep going? What are you trying to prove? Maybe you're like some women: the ones who keep going because once they've set a goal, nothing—not even pregnancy—is going to keep them from meeting it. Or the ones who want to take as little time off from running as possible to maintain fitness. Or others who simply seek bragging rights: "I ran until the day he was born."

My reasons included some of the above and a few others, like wanting to be able to explain to readers what 9 months of running feels like, justifying my expensive maternity running tights, and placing faith in a study that said exercise would trim a few days off my pregnancy. (I delivered both my sons before their due dates, though many of the runners interviewed for this book were not so lucky.)

Labor of Love?

By now you know that running will give you a healthier pregnancy and a speedier return to your pre-pregnancy fitness level. But will it help you during actual labor? Unfortunately, research doesn't provide any definitive answers. Some studies show that exercise shaves a few days off pregnancy; others show that it doesn't. Some researchers have discovered that women who exercise during pregnancy have shorter labors; others have discovered just the opposite.

Here's the good news: Most exercise and pregnancy research concurs when it comes to what kind of delivery you might have. Women who exercise during pregnancy are less likely to need a cesarean than nonexercisers and are also less likely to require intervention with forceps or vacuum extractors.

The bottom line? Don't get your hopes up for a shorter pregnancy and easier delivery just because you dragged yourself off the couch every day. Do take comfort in the fact that you're healthier and fitter than moms who didn't.

Try to understand your own reasons, not only so that you can answer your mother-in-law when she quizzes you for the 40th time, but so that you know yourself. It will be easier to get out the door during these last few weeks if you can remind yourself why you're doing it in the first place. And you will be a stronger runner and a stronger person if you appreciate the motivation that kept you running all this way.

The Nesting Instinct

You may have thought people were kidding when they described the nesting instinct, but it creeps up on most pregnant women before they realize it's unnecessary to stack soup cans in alphabetical order or repaint the guest room closet.

Go ahead and give in to the craziness if you're pursuing something worthwhile, especially if it benefits the baby or will make your life easier after he's born. But if you're obsessing, give it up and do something purely for yourself—go to a movie, get a massage, have a pedicure. You won't have much time for that kind of thing after the baby is born.

More Fun with Leaking

It's not bad enough that your bladder may leak; your breasts may get into the act, too. Colostrum (or pre-milk) can build up in your breasts during the last couple months of pregnancy and let loose in trickles or drops. Most women don't have this problem, but just in case, keep some nursing pads on hand to tuck in to your running bra. (You'll need them later anyway if you're going to breastfeed.) Nursing pads are thin cotton circles about the size of a silver-dollar pancake. With all the compression in your bra these days, you should have no problem keeping them in place.

A much more serious type of leaking is the bloody kind that may appear on your underwear. Consider it an emergency if your blood is bright red because it could mean that the blood is coming from the placenta and may indicate a threat to your baby. Even if it's more like brown spotting or mucus with pink, brown, or red streaks, it's worth a call to the doctor just to rule out any problems. Bloody mucus accompanied by strong contractions at regular intervals means that your labor has started. Contact your doctor right away.

Finally . . . diarrhea. Although this might seem like a foreign concept after so many months of fighting constipation, diarrhea is actually a good sign that labor will start within a few hours. Speed-dial your doc.

YOUR CONCERNS

False Labor

Was ever a crueler term invented than *false labor*? Your body can actually trick you into thinking the baby is coming when it has no intention of producing him anytime soon! You're left making exasperated explanations after the hospital sends you home bitter and pregnant. It's probably not real labor if:

- Your contractions don't involve your lower back.

- Your contractions aren't at regular intervals and don't increase over time.

- Your contractions ease when you move around.

- You are spotting brownish blood (indicating cervical bleeding) but are not feeling contractions.

If you have any doubts, call your doctor. It's better to embarrass yourself out of caution than to give birth someplace you didn't intend to.

Overdue Baby

Your doctor considers your due date an estimate of when your baby will be born. You can't help but see it as a guarantee. So if you're one of the 50 percent of women who stay pregnant past their due dates, you probably feel a bit disappointed. And if you're one of the very few pregnant women still running, you possess some considerable bragging rights.

Fortunately, most doctors will induce you if you go more than a week past your due date because the quality of the placenta can start to deteriorate. Don't fall prey to the myth that an induced labor hurts more than a natural one. All labor hurts. If it becomes too much, you can ask for pain medication.

Real Labor

If you're still running as you near your due date, run closer to home in case contractions start or your water breaks. Do half-mile loops around your neighborhood or run up and down your street. Let your husband, a friend, or a neighbor know you're leaving for your run and make sure he or she will be near the phone in case of emergency.

As you run, pay attention to any unusual sensations. Geri Sorenson, a runner and mother of five from Kildeer, Illinois, felt her first contractions while running. "They felt like a side ache, which I never get, so I stopped and walked," she says. "After I showered and changed, my

(continued on page 186)

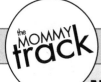

NO REST FOR THE PREGNANT

Name: Nora Tobin
Birth date: November 1967
Residence: Anchorage
Occupation: University instructor
Children: Two, born 1999 and 2002

PREGNANCY ROCKS

Ask Nora Tobin to recount her athletic accomplishments and she may be hard-pressed to remember them all. She's conquered everything from the international Eco-Challenge (twice) to local trail races in the mountains near her home in Anchorage, where she frequently sets the course record. She is as well-known in the climbing community and on the cross-country ski circuit as she is among runners.

In fact, it was while on a 4-day climb in Yosemite National Park that she got the initial clue she was pregnant with her firstborn. "Usually when I do these multi-day climbing routes, I'm not hungry because I'm so focused," she says. "I was insanely hungry up there. I kept trading my water for food."

Once back in Anchorage, she confirmed that she was expecting and located a midwife who would support her athletic endeavors during pregnancy. "Her philosophy is, 'If it doesn't hurt and you don't bleed, you can do it,'" says Nora. (It's especially hard to find medical professionals who allow rock climbing. And for good reason: Unless you're as skilled and fit as Nora, you should stay off sheer rock faces when you're pregnant.)

Throughout both her pregnancies, Nora continued to climb at a rock gym twice a week. She ran through her fifth month and replaced that with cross-country skiing when the snow came. "I always try to take time off from running in the winter," she says. "It gives my body a break."

Not that she didn't ski hard. At 7½ months into her second pregnancy, she joined the annual Tour of Anchorage 50-K ski race and placed in the top 20. "I looked very pregnant," she says. "I got a lot of cheering from the crowd."

Fittingly, Nora was skiing a mountain trail during her second pregnancy when her water broke. She assumed she was experiencing more of the stress incontinence that had sometimes bothered her since the first pregnancy. By the time she realized she was in labor, summoned her husband on the cell phone, and reached the birthing center, she had an hour to spare.

HAVE FAMILY, WILL RACE

Nora began working out again within 3 weeks of her first delivery and 2 weeks of her second. Though running and skiing in between breast-feeding was tricky, she managed. "My husband would say, 'Ready . . . go!' and I'd hurry out and ski or do a trail run, and try to get back before the baby started crying." The physical and emotional boost was worth the exhaustion. And her efforts paid off. Two months after her first child's birth, she placed third in a 5-K trail race with a 3,000-foot elevation gain. And she came in second in a 14-mile mountain race with a 9,000-foot elevation gain just 10 weeks after giving birth the second time.

Her next challenge will be the annual Hardrock Hundred Mile Endurance Run in Colorado, an event that takes 2 days to complete. Nora will train for the race at altitude when the Tobin family temporarily relocates to Colorado for her husband's teaching sabbatical.

NORA'S TIPS

Run with your friends. "They can tie your shoes for you when you're too big to bend over. Try not to get depressed if you can't keep up."

Throw away your watch. "That way you won't get uptight about your sluggish time."

Wear a really good bra. "I wore one, through my pregnancy and afterward, called the Corset. It had at least 20 little snaps and held everything in place, especially during the time I was breastfeeding. Double bras don't work when you're really, really big."

Subdued Movements

If your little wiggler seems less wiggly these days, you really can't blame him. Quarters are tight. One friend of mine claimed that she could identify her baby's body parts—elbows, knees, bottom—through her own belly. Babies tend to roll rather than kick during the ninth month. The quality of the movement is less important than the quantity (unless the movement appears frantic, which could indicate lack of oxygen, in which case you should call the doctor).

If you're concerned that your baby hasn't been moving often enough, lie down and try to count 10 movements within 1 hour. Once you lie still and concentrate, you'll probably notice the baby's minor shifts and changes more readily. If you don't count 10 movements within 1 hour, contact your doctor right away.

water broke." Sorenson's experience didn't fit the classic labor symptoms, probably because she was in the middle of a run and interpreted them as a running-related ache.

If you feel a contraction during your run, one that hurts enough to make you stop, walk home, lie down, and begin timing your contractions. "If you're bleeding or your water breaks, call for help right away," says Patty Kulpa, M.D., a sports gynecologist from Gig Harbor, Washington.

Normally, you can count on one or more indicators to let you know labor has arrived. Call your doctor if you experience any of the following:

- You have contractions that are difficult to talk through and come at regular intervals 5 to 7 minutes apart (or less).

- Contractions intensify when you move around.

- Contractions begin coming at more frequent intervals.

- You feel pain that includes your lower back and feels like menstrual cramps.

- Amniotic fluid leaks from your vagina in either a trickle or a gush, indicating that your water has broken. This feels a little like peeing, but most women can tell the difference—unless it happens while they sleep. Call your doctor immediately.

Nothing is more exciting than the beginning of labor. Even though you know it's going to hurt, you can't wait to be done with pregnancy and meet the baby. After all these months of imagining what he will look like, you're finally going to get to see for yourself.

First you have work to do. The first stage of labor, during which your cervix dilates, includes three phases. The early phase, when your cervix opens to 5 centimeters, is pretty much a cakewalk. (Some women don't even realize they're in labor at this point.) The contractions feel no worse than bad menstrual cramps, and possibly the worst part is knowing that things will become a whole lot more painful soon. Your doctor will tell you whether you should stay home or head to the hospital during this part of labor.

The second, or active, phase hurts—think menstrual cramps powered by electricity. Your cervix opens to 8 centimeters. Many women

Why Your Marathon Doesn't Matter

When I ran my first marathon 2½ years before delivering my first child, I thought, "All this pain is good preparation for childbirth."

I was sadly mistaken. Endurance is the only thing these events have in common. Very little else is even similar. For one thing, pushing—the most memorable part of labor—is much closer to strength training than to running. When you push, you use every muscle in your body to force the baby out. Unlike a marathon, there's no FINISH banner rippling in the distance. Once labor starts, you know it will end—you just have no idea when. And you can't bail from labor. There's no sag vehicle to pick you up if you quit.

On a positive note, the prize at the end of labor and delivery is way better than any race T-shirt, even the long-sleeve ones.

ask for an epidural during this phase, which is a good time to do so because the pain will only get worse.

During the third, or transition, phase, the contractions get more intense as they work to dilate your cervix to the full 10 centimeters and move you into the second stage of labor: pushing.

Pushing is the stage that produces the most childbirth stories. It will tax you beyond belief. Every muscle in your body will strain as you work to expel the baby. After it's over, in addition to smarting from your pelvic floor injuries, you may feel sore in your back, arms, and legs.

The final stage, when the placenta emerges, is forgettable. After the trauma your vagina and pelvic floor muscles have just experienced—and the distraction caused by your new baby—you'll barely notice passing the placenta.

Delivery

The moment you've both feared and yearned for has arrived: Your baby is passing through the birth canal (or abdomen if you are having a C-section) and out of your body. No matter how tired you are, listen to your doctor's instructions. Adhering to them could mean the difference between tearing your perineum and not. Your doctor may want to perform an episiotomy (an incision in your perineum) to enlarge your vaginal opening. It's a good idea to have discussed this with her prior to labor, especially if you hope to avoid one. This surgical procedure—used routinely just a few years ago—is a hot topic these days. It creates more room for the baby to exit the body but is scary for the woman and takes time to heal. That may mean a longer wait before returning to running.

If you're so inclined, go ahead and watch your baby being born. All you have to do is lift your head up and you'll never see anything more amazing. (During a C-section, a nurse will block your belly with a sterile sheet to shield you from seeing the incision as it is made. Ask to have it lowered slightly as the baby emerges.) Don't be disappointed

Going Natural

The type of childbirth you choose—medicated or natural—may affect how quickly you return to running after your baby is born. Studies show that pain medication, namely the epidural, can result in longer labor and an increased need for the use of forceps or vacuum extraction. Both can cause additional tearing, and forceps deliveries usually require an episiotomy.

A medicated delivery probably means a longer recovery time for you and a longer layoff from running. Besides your desire to run again, there are other reasons to deliver naturally, including wanting your baby to be free of medication in his bloodstream. For some women, it's even a financial call. My friend Kelly Gerlach, a runner and mother of three from Gakona, Alaska, refused an epidural during her second and third deliveries. "It's not worth the copayment," she says. "I'd rather put it toward a mountain bike." Which she did with no regrets.

But you don't need to be a hero. If you want pain medication, ask for it. In the grand scheme of things, a few extra days or weeks off from running isn't going to hurt you.

if you aren't instantly flooded with motherly love. You may be too wiped out to appreciate it, but later you'll be glad you saw the first moments of your child's life.

Having a Cesarean

If life were fair, all C-sections would be scheduled in advance. As it stands, many women who end up giving birth by cesarean have to endure labor first. That means a double whammy—hard labor followed by hard recovery.

Most unplanned surgical deliveries aren't considered an emergency. Your doctor will perform an emergency C-section if your baby's life or long-term health (or yours) is in danger. Typically you'll be sedated with general anesthesia. Your doctor may make a vertical incision in your abdomen; it's a faster procedure than making a horizontal incision but takes longer to heal.

In the case of a scheduled or unplanned nonemergency C-section, you'll likely be given a regional anesthetic, such as an epidural or spinal block, to numb your lower body. A catheter will be inserted into your bladder to keep it drained and out of the doctor's way. Then the doctor will make a small "bikini" incision in the skin in your lower abdomen, followed by a deeper incision into the uterus. The doctor will lift your baby out and let you get a look at him before handing him to a nurse. Finally, the doctor will remove the placenta and sew you up. Altogether, a C-section takes about 30 minutes, including about 5 minutes for the actual birth.

Some women perceive having a cesarean as a failure, as if delivering vaginally were a prerequisite for motherhood. Athletes can be particularly susceptible to this notion because some consider vaginal childbirth as a chance to put their athletic skills to the test. Upon having her cesarean, my friend Catherine Plichta, a Richmond, Virginia, athlete and mother of two, felt dismayed. "My second child was breech and I had to have a C-section. It really threw me because I'd been thinking, 'I'm in such great shape; this baby's going to go flying across the room.'" As Catherine concluded after her daughter was born, the method is much less important than the outcome. "Your athletic ability doesn't matter," she says. "What matters is a healthy baby."

CHAPTER 14

THE "FOURTH" TRIMESTER

RUNNING AND BEYOND

SOMEDAY YOU'LL LOOK BACK on your baby's first days and forget what your body is going through right now. The extent of damage to your vagina and surrounding areas (or your abdomen if you had a C-section) is truly mind-boggling. You knew it would be bad, but no one told you there would be this much blood and swelling. (And let's face it, would you have wanted to know?) Childbirth is an amazing study in contrasts: joy, pain, fear, hope. Fortunately the joy and the hope affix themselves in our memories, and eventually we overlook the injuries we sustained giving birth.

Your body is working diligently to repair all the damage, and considering what it's been through, it does a fine job. The best thing you can do as a woman, a mother, and a runner is take care of yourself. Eat well, drink lots of fluids, sleep whenever you can, and take advantage of the kindness of obstetrical nurses. You're not a bad mother if you ask the nurses to take your baby to the nursery if she prevents you from sleeping. Your job is to go home as rested and recovered as possible so that you can be a good mother.

Above all, don't do anything foolish like trying to exercise vigorously. Even slogging through the maternity ward corridors isn't a good idea. If the hospital offers whirlpool or sitz baths, use them as much as you're allowed—unless of course you're too busy sleeping.

If you've chosen to breastfeed, work hard to establish a good connection with your baby. Breastfeeding a baby is a time-consuming endeavor—even more so if it doesn't come naturally. Rely on the lactation consultant in the hospital. The sooner you and your baby are in sync, the sooner breastfeeding will become a normal, comfortable part of life and the sooner you'll have control of your time again. That should mean an easier transition back to running.

RECOVERY

Going Home

Getting ready to leave the hospital may be a pitifully slow process, since you've probably spent most of your time in bed caring for yourself and your baby and very little time staying organized. Unless your husband or birth partner has kept your hospital bag in order, you'll need to repack, making sure to locate all the personal items you've sprinkled around the room. Then there are the armloads of "freebies" the hospital gives you and the bouquets of flowers that friends and family have sent.

Because of your injuries, showering takes extra time, and you may need assistance if you feel weak. Budget twice the time it normally takes, and if you're planning your regular beauty routine afterward, expect to take breaks. Just standing at the mirror and fiddling with your hair for a few minutes can make you dizzy and queasy.

Allow plenty of time to feed and change the baby before you go home—it usually takes longer than you expect. And try not to become frustrated with the slow pace. It will continue for a few weeks until you heal and become more adept at handling your newborn.

Comfort tip: Before you leave, ask the nurse if she can give you extra ice packs. Hospitals often use chemical ones that become cold

After Birth

Your body will start healing noticeably 2 to 3 days postpartum. Some of the bleeding will taper off and turn brownish. Your skin may have a corpselike pallor, most noticeably on your face. Your breasts may appear gigantic if your milk has come in, and if you're breastfeeding, your nipples may look and feel raw.

If you look in the mirror before showering, you'll be amazed at the state of your abdomen. For one thing, you won't be ready for your pre-pregnancy jeans just yet—you'll still look about 4 months pregnant. Your belly may appear wrinkly and feel stretchy, and your linea nigra ("ripe stripe") will contrast sharply with your skin, like ink on a deflated birthday balloon.

With luck, there's one difference between you and a new mother who didn't run through her pregnancy: Your weight may be closer to what it was pre-pregnancy. Some new moms who ran during those 9 months find themselves within 4 to 6 pounds of their pre-pregnancy weight. (Don't sweat it if you're not. Those jeans will fit soon enough.)

when you bend them and crack their inner core. These ice packs will continue to soothe your swollen perineum once you're home.

Your Emotions

After the humbling experience of giving birth, you'll undertake the equally humbling experience of new motherhood. You may question every decision and worry that you have done/are doing/will do something to harm the baby. You'll wear down the redial button on your phone with repeated calls to your child's pediatrician over things like umbilical cord stumps, circumcisions, and perpetual crying.

Your mind may be on the birth itself, especially if it didn't meet your expectations. Perhaps you weren't expecting that C-section, forceps delivery, or medical student observer. Or maybe you just wish the whole experience hadn't been so far beyond your control. (We runners are known for our love of control, by the way.)

You may be frustrated by the stop/start nature of your body's recovery. Some days will be better than others, and some days it may feel like you're back to square one. Your return to running may seem light years away.

Sleep deprivation and hormonal changes fuel your emotions as your body tries to regain its balance. This doesn't make your feelings less valid. Talk to a friend who has been through childbirth to gain some perspective. If this doesn't help, find a counselor who specializes in postpartum issues.

Talk to your husband, too. He's probably worried about the baby and about you, since he witnessed what you went through. Talk about your individual styles of baby care so that you understand and respect your differences. Agree on a schedule that allows each of you to rest (although your rest should get priority, since your body is recovering from major injuries).

Postpartum Depression

Postpartum depression is a feeling of hopelessness that strikes some women in the weeks and months after they give birth. No one knows the precise cause, but hormone changes seem to be the main physiological culprit, with exhaustion, caring for a newborn, and isolation as some of the accomplices. Symptoms include:

- Inability to concentrate

- Insomnia

- Loss of appetite

- Feeling like a failure

- Severe mood swings

- Thoughts of suicide and death

- Fear of harming the baby

- Inability to make decisions

- Panic

You might recognize a few of these even if you don't suffer from full-blown postpartum depression. About 60 to 80 percent of new mothers experience a less severe version of it called *baby blues*. It develops within a few hours to a few days of delivering and usually resolves on its own within a week or two.

If you feel depressed, you can try to alleviate it on your own. Here's how.

Ask for help. Your family and friends can help with cooking, housework, and child care. Sometimes it's daunting to ask, especially when you already feel unsure of yourself, but try to muster the courage.

Call your friends to talk. You might have to preface the conversation with "Can I whine for a few minutes?" Anyone who's been home with a newborn will know why you're asking.

Recovery Advice from Running Moms

"Take it slowly and keep hydrated. Stop and walk if you feel uncomfortable. Don't let your mind overrule what your body is telling you."

—*Geri Sorenson, Kildeer, Illinois*

"Now is the time to take care of the baby. This isn't the time to do something crazy."

— *Linda Gill, San Anselmo, California*

"Don't be impatient and push yourself too hard. Patience is the hardest part. You'll get there."

—*Lynda Del Missier, Tampa, Florida*

"Let your body heal. It's just done an incredible feat."

— *Shannon Avery, Puerto Rico*

"Women are not socialized to meet their needs first. Tell your partner you need to run. Happy mom, happy baby. In fact, happy mom, happy family."

— *Nora Tobin, Anchorage, Alaska*

Try to get some sleep. That means squeezing it in whenever you can, day or night. Once you've gotten a little rest, try to find some personal time. Sometimes a 20-minute nap followed by 20 minutes of reading or a hobby can do the trick.

Eat well. Take advantage of the casseroles and dinners that friends or neighbors drop off. Make sure your kitchen stays stocked with fruits, veggies, and healthy snacks. Soup and sandwich combinations make quick, nutritious meals. Give your husband a grocery list so that he can shop on his way home from work. Or ask a friend to do it for a couple of weeks until you recuperate.

Exercise if you can. Exercise can have an antidepressant effect, says Frank Webbe, Ph.D., professor of psychology at Florida Institute of Technology in Melbourne and president of a group called the Running Psychologists. "And it's quicker than drugs or psychotherapy."

If you can't exercise, don't worry. Too much pressure to run or exercise might make you feel like even more of a failure or more overwhelmed. "People with depression have trouble doing anything, let alone exercising," says Judy Van Raalte, Ph.D., a runner, mother of two, and professor of psychology at Springfield College in Massachusetts. Rely on the other suggestions above to get you back on track.

If nothing works or you feel like you can't bring yourself to do any of these, call your obstetrician. She may want to see you, or she may give you a referral. Chances are good that she'll know a therapist who specializes in postpartum depression. Treatment will probably include psychotherapy and antidepressant medication, although it may vary based on your preferences, the doctor's preferences, and the severity of your depression.

Resting and Walking When You'd Rather Run

In its quest to return to normal, your body may make you crazy. You might sweat for no apparent reason and urinate copiously while your body tries to rid itself of excess fluids. Your hormones will fluctuate, as will your body temperature. You may get up from your cozy bed for a feeding and shiver uncontrollably. If this happens, cuddle with your baby and wrap up in as many blankets as you can find. Your uterus may contract as it shrinks back to normal, causing cramps. (This happens more frequently during breastfeeding.) If you have stitches from tearing or an episiotomy, they may sting and later itch. Sitz baths work well for both problems.

As soon as you sense the slightest return to normal in your body, you'll start thinking about running again. Most pregnancy books suggest that you wait until after your 6-week checkup to exercise strenuously. But healing, like childbirth, is an individual matter. Some women feel ready to run within a few days of a vaginal delivery, some not until 6 weeks. "After my first baby, I went running a week after delivery," says Joy Gayter, a Lake Bluff, Illinois, runner and mother of three. "I felt like my insides were coming out. With my second, I waited 2 weeks. And with my third, I was much smarter and waited 6 weeks." If you and your doctor haven't already discussed when you can return to running, give her a call before you try it.

The best indicator of whether you've started back too soon is bleeding. If you come home to find bright red blood on your pad, lie down for 30 minutes and take off another 2 or 3 days before you try again. You must listen to and respect your body. Your injuries will heal more quickly when you take good care of yourself.

Walking can help alleviate your frustration, but sometimes even this can cause you to bleed. Try slowing down, even if it means barely moving. Just a little forward motion can help you feel better emotionally as you wait out your recovery.

GETTING BACK ON TRACK

Running Again

When you no longer bleed bright red, begin to add some running to your walking routine—assuming you've already secured your doctor's permission. "Start slowly, like after you've been injured," says Lisa Keller, an Anchorage, Alaska, triathlete and mother of two. Begin with a combination of running and walking, as outlined in the program below.

After the first 6 weeks of running, continue adding 1 to 5 minutes a week to the running portion and allow ample time to walk, which

6 Weeks to Running Again

	WEEK 1	WEEK 2	WEEK 3
Day 1	Walk 10 min; run 1 min; walk 5 min; run 1 min; walk 5 min; run 1 min; walk 2 min (Total: 25 min)	Rest	Walk 10 min; run 17 min; walk 10 min (Total: 37 min)
Day 2	Walk 10 min; run 2 min; walk 4 min; run 2 min; walk 4 min; run 2 min; walk 2 min (Total: 26 min)	Walk 10 min; run 10 min; walk 10 min (Total: 30 min)	Walk 10 min; run 18 min; walk 10 min (Total: 38 min)
Day 3	Rest	Walk 10 min; run 10 min; walk 10 min (Total: 30 min)	Rest
Day 4	Walk 10 min; run 2 min; walk 4 min; run 2 min; walk 4 min; run 2 min; walk 2 min (Total: 26 min)	Rest	Walk 10 min; run 20 min; walk 10 min (Total: 40 min)
Day 5	Walk 10 min; run 2 min; walk 4 min; run 2 min; walk 4 min; run 2 min; walk 2 min (Total: 26 min)	Walk 10 min; run 15 min; walk 10 min (Total: 35 min)	Walk 10 min; run 20 min; walk 10 min (Total: 40 min)
Day 6	Rest	Walk 10 min; run 15 min; walk 10 min (Total: 35 min)	Walk 10 min; run 20 min; walk 10 min (Total: 40 min)
Day 7	Walk 10 min; run 10 min; walk 10 min (Total: 30 min)	Rest	Walk 10 min; run 20 min; walk 10 min (Total: 40 min)

warms up your muscles. Cool down for at least 5 minutes by jogging or walking.

Feel free to modify the program given here or ignore it altogether. You know your body better than anyone else. Just try to be patient in your exuberance. Here are tips for a successful return to running.

	WEEK 4	WEEK 5	WEEK 6
Day 1	Walk 10 min; run 20 min; walk 10 min (Total: 40 min)	Rest	Walk 7 min; run 30 min; walk 5 min (Total: 42 min)
Day 2	Rest	Walk 10 min; run 25 min; walk 5 min (Total: 40 min)	Walk 7 min; run 30 min; walk 5 min (Total: 42 min)
Day 3	Walk 10 min; run 22 min; walk 10 min (Total: 42 min)	Walk 10 min; run 25 min; walk 5 min (Total: 40 min)	Rest
Day 4	Walk 10 min; run 22 min; walk 10 min (Total: 42 min)	Rest	Walk 7 min; run 30 min; walk 5 min (Total: 42 min)
Day 5	Rest	Walk 10 min; run 27 min; walk 5 min (Total: 42 min)	Walk 7 min; run 30 min; walk 5 min (Total: 42 min)
Day 6	Rest	Walk 10 min; run 27 min; walk 5 min (Total: 42 min)	Rest
Day 7	Walk 10 min; run 23 min; walk 10 min (Total: 43 min)	Rest	Walk 7 min; run 32 min; walk 5 min (Total: 44 min)

- Plan your running into your day, but be flexible. The baby's needs may preempt your scheduled run, so identify several possible time slots just in case.

- Keep your expectations realistic. Respect the toll that pregnancy and childbirth have taken on your body.

- Eat 1 to 2 hours before your workout or carry a gel pack or other high-glycemic snack. (This is especially pertinent to nursing moms.)

- Drink enough fluid so that your urine runs pale (also extra important for nursing moms).

- Reevaluate your running bras. If you're nursing, you may need to increase another size or double up.

- Stop if you feel sharp pain in your perineum, abdomen, breasts, or anywhere else. Call the doctor if pain persists.

- Don't run if you have an infection of the breast or reproductive organs.

- Ignore your pace for the first 3 months of running.

- Don't be a slave to the bathroom scale. Your weight will fluctuate in the first 2 to 3 months as your body strives to find its equilibrium.

- If running drains your energy, cut back mileage or take extra rest days.

No matter when you resume your training, consider the combination of efforts your body is making. First, it's recovering from delivery; second, it's readjusting to running; and third, it's using muscles you never thought you had as you haul around the baby—sometimes in a heavy car seat. New moms can get themselves into weird positions, resulting in all kinds of back problems, says Patty Kulpa, M.D., a sports gynecologist from Gig Harbor, Washington.

Only one of the runners interviewed for this book injured herself during pregnancy, but several did soon after. "After my second child, I didn't pay much attention to my body as I was running," says Blythe Marston, an Anchorage runner and mother of two. "I waited 10 days after my baby was born, and 6 weeks later I was running about 2 hours.

Running after a Cesarean

You won't be standing in front of a mirror 2 days after having a C-section. In fact, you'll probably spend a full 4 days in the hospital. Since you've just undergone major abdominal surgery *and* given birth, you'll feel pain from both sides of the equation. Your incision will hurt and you may feel nausea, gas pains, and even shoulder pain (referred from your diaphragm, which often becomes irritated) as a result of surgery. As after a vaginal delivery, your uterus will contract as it returns to its normal size, causing you to feel crampy. (You will need to use sanitary pads for a couple of weeks while your uterus heals and expels the material built up during your pregnancy.)

For at least the first 2 to 3 weeks after you get home, you'll probably be bed- or couch-ridden most of the time. Advice varies on when you can return to running, but the main indicator is how you feel. "I went jogging again for the first time when my daughter was 4 weeks, and it hurt," says my friend Catherine Plichta, a Richmond, Virginia, athlete and mother of two. "It wasn't the incision on the outside that hurt. It was deep inside. So I waited another 2 weeks and then started back."

Once you get your doctor's okay, run on flat surfaces at first to avoid irritating your incision, suggests Patty Kulpa, M.D., a sports gynecologist from Gig Harbor, Washington. "Start with walking, then work into a brisk walk, and then into jogging. After that, go by your pain. Don't push it, especially for the first couple of weeks after you've started back."

One day my right hamstring just started freezing up. I spent 5 weeks trying to figure out what was going on."

Anchorage triathlete Lisa Keller competed hard in a sprint triathlon 5 months after having her first baby. "It wasn't necessarily the distance," she says. "It was the intensity of the work I was doing. I did too much too fast, and I started having hip problems."

Give yourself a reality check: Are you running too hard or too fast? You know your body and your history best. If you've been prone to overdoing it in the past, you probably will now. It's hard to curb your excitement at returning to running, especially after the bleeding stops and your body feels somewhat normal again. One of the biggest "danger zones" is the period from 6 weeks to 3 months postpartum. Runners typically ignore the little pains nagging at them, yet these can easily escalate into full-scale injuries. Cut back or cross-train if something hurts.

If you injure yourself now, you may risk repeated problems long after your child is in preschool.

Incontinence Revisited

Whether or not you leaked urine during pregnancy, you may leak postpartum, especially when you run, cough, or even laugh. Most women with urinary incontinence experience a small trickle that can be soaked up by an ordinary sanitary pad. In the meantime, keep doing those Kegels. For the exercises to be effective, you need to practice them three to four times a week. Each session should contain about 10 repetitions of holding to your maximum ability for 8 to 10 seconds (lasting about 5 minutes total). "One of the reasons Kegels aren't always effective is that people think they should help in 2 weeks, so they quit," says Ingrid Nygaard, M.D., an associate professor of obstetrics and gynecology at the University of Iowa. "It takes a good 2 to 3 months before people start to notice improvement for stress incontinence."

Once your incontinence is under control, continue the exercises at least three times a week, and don't just practice. Apply Kegels to your everyday life—contracting your PC muscles, say, before you jump or cough so that you don't experience incontinence during those times. Performing Kegels is a lifelong process, says Dr. Nygaard. Just like your leg muscles get out of shape when you don't run, your pelvic floor muscles get out of shape when you don't work them.

Aside from performing Kegels, watch your fluid intake. Caffeine can exacerbate stress incontinence if you drink three or more cups of coffee (or the equivalent) a day. Some doctors also suspect that artificial sweeteners, carbonated beverages, and alcohol contribute to the problem. Try eliminating these substances for a few days to see if continence returns. If bladder control does not improve within 6 months—or if it's more like a gush than a trickle—contact your doctor.

The Incontinence Secret

As I'm sure you've learned by now, your friends and doctors haven't told you everything there is to know about pregnancy and postpartum experiences. You probably don't want to know everything anyway—it will just cause more anxiety. However, there is something to be said for being prepared, especially as a runner. So I give you this information: During delivery, you can damage your anal sphincter muscle, the nerves to the muscle, or both. As a result, you may release stool and/or gas when you don't intend to. It's called *fecal incontinence*. Some women are too embarrassed to report it, even to their doctors.

There's no need for shame. About 5 percent of women who deliver vaginally end up with this problem. If the damage is to your sphincter muscle (and doesn't include nerves), surgery can often repair the problem. If you did sustain nerve damage during delivery and it can't be fixed, your doctor may be able to help you manage the incontinence. You might think running is out of the question, but a few key strategies will help you stay on the road.

- Since most people lose only liquid stools, it pays to "bulk up." Take a fiber supplement like Metamucil or FiberCon, but with minimal fluids. This will help harden stools.

- Take an antidiarrhea medicine like Imodium about 1 hour before your run.

- Keep track of the foods that worsen your incontinence and avoid them.

- Develop healthy bowel habits. Try to have one bowel movement every morning instead of several little ones. To accomplish this, take advantage of a natural reflex that triggers a bowel movement 15 to 30 minutes after breakfast, says Ingrid Nygaard, M.D., associate professor of obstetrics and gynecology at the University of Iowa. "For most women, if they've already had their good bowel movement, then they don't have stool sitting in the rectum waiting to come out, and they're not going to leak with running."

A very common cause of fecal incontinence is irritable bowel syndrome, which has nothing to do with your delivery. If you alternate between constipation and diarrhea and if you feel abdominal cramping, mention it to your doctor. Medication and lifestyle changes can alleviate it.

Feeding Yourself

Even without a baby inside, you still need to nourish your body well. "A new mom needs calories to recover," says Nancy Clark, R.D., author of *Nancy Clark's Sports Nutrition Guidebook* and a nutrition counselor at SportsMedicine Associates in Brookline, Massachusetts. Eat the right combinations of wholesome foods to get a balance of carbohydrates, protein, and fat, she says. Some examples include cereal, milk, and a banana; bread, peanut butter, and yogurt; and spaghetti, tomato sauce, and meatballs. Breastfeeding requires about 500 extra calories a day, and now that you're running again, you'll need another 100 calories per mile.

Drink plenty of fluids especially if you're breastfeeding. Again, your urine should be clear and you should be making regular visits to the toilet.

Feeding the Baby

Breastfeeding and running both draw on your body's hydration levels. Set water bottles and juice boxes around the house in your favorite nursing spots so that you'll always have something to drink. Don't leave for a run without a water bottle. In fact, don't leave home at all without a water bottle. Keep the baby's diaper bag stocked for your needs, too.

Choose a running bra that doesn't chafe your breasts or cause further soreness to your nipples. Take it off as soon as you can after working out. If you leaked milk into your bra or nursing pads and it dried, check whether the fabric is stuck to your skin. If it is, moisten the fabric with warm water before you pull it off. Avoid your nipples when you lather up in the shower; the soap can further dry and irritate them.

If you bottlefeed your baby, you'll have a little more freedom than nursing moms. A father or other caregiver can feed the baby anytime she's hungry, which means you can get out for a run more easily. Also, formula often satisfies the baby for longer—3 to 4 hours instead of 2 or 2½.

You may have less trouble staying hydrated than breastfeeding moms, although you should still pay close attention to the color and volume of your urine, since sleep deprivation, recovery, and running draw plenty from your body's water stores.

Stock your freezer with bags of frozen vegetables so that you can ice your breasts when the milk comes in, around 3 days postpartum. They'll alleviate much of the engorgement pain, and you can use them again if you have running sore spots or injuries. Aspirin and ibuprofen also help with engorgement pain.

Run on Empty

If you are breastfeeding, coordinating your baby's feedings and your running can feel daunting at first. Milk-laden breasts are heavy and cumbersome, so feed first, then run. Understand that your plans to hit the trail by a certain time will evaporate if your baby dawdles or needs extra comfort, so be flexible.

If you have to run first and nurse afterward, ignore the stories about babies not accepting postexercise breast milk because of higher lactic acid levels. That's old news. Several recent studies show that babies readily accept their mother's milk after she has exercised.

Running with Baby— Again

There you go again, running with the baby sticking way out in front of you. This time she's in a stroller, and your running life is far more comfortable than it was when you were pregnant. Running with a stroller is not entirely without complications, but it gives you one more way to carry on.

Wait until your baby can control her head well and her pediatrician okays it before you put her in the running stroller—usually at about 6 months. Bundle her up in cool weather, and don't take her out when it's very cold; the breeze created by your forward motion will chill her even further. Keep the sun out of her eyes, protect her skin with sunscreen, and don't run with her when it's very hot.

(continued on page 208)

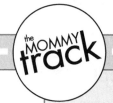

KEEPING A BALANCE

Name: Kristin Alexander

Birth date: February 1968

Residence: Chicago

Occupation: Social worker

Children: Two, born 1998 and 2001

STAYING SANE

For Kristin Alexander, running is all about balance. Not the kind that saves you from canting sideways with your big belly but the kind that keeps you sane in the midst of chaos. As a crisis social worker in an emergency room, Kristin's professional life carries an intensity most of us can't imagine. Add two kids and a husband who works full-time, and things quickly can feel out of control. "I run as much for mental or emotional reasons as I do for physical reasons," she says.

Pregnancy slowed Kristin but didn't stop her. She cut her 25 miles a week in half, and she consciously slowed her pace to avoid overexerting herself. During her first trimesters of both pregnancies, she felt dog-tired and nauseated much of the time. "I would get up and run first thing in the morning," she says, "so I didn't have time to think about it."

Kristin describes both her pregnancies as easy, the second even more so than the first. For some unknown reason, the second pregnancy seemed to take a lighter toll on her bladder, so she didn't have to make frequent pit stops. That meant she could run farther into that pregnancy (6½ months rather than 5). The emotional side was easier, too. "With the second one, you're used to having your life kind of chaotic. You don't have the luxury to be tired all the time."

Kristin balanced out her running with walking, water aerobics, and yoga. "The water aerobics class was great because I felt like I was my normal weight," she says. Prenatal yoga was not strenuous, so it gave her time each week to focus on the baby and be excited about the pregnancy.

TIMING IT RIGHT

Three weeks after delivering her second baby, Kristin was on the trail again. "I healed really quickly that time," she says. (She had waited 6 weeks after her first baby.) Her running felt good, and the only real challenge was coordinating her workouts with breast-feeding. "You have to time it so you feed the baby and get out right away before the milk comes in again," she says. She learned that the hard way one day when she stayed out with her running buddies a bit too long. "I was engorged, so I knew the baby was hungry," she says. "And I had to run home with huge breasts."

MIXING IT UP

Within a few months of giving birth to her second child, Kristin set her sights on the LaSalle Bank Chicago Marathon. And 18 months postpartum, she completed it in 4:29. But training made her feel burned out and out of balance, so she mixed things up. She joined a health club that offers free child care, and she added a new training element: "I take a ballet class twice a week. And I still run two mornings a week. Now I'm having fun."

KRISTIN'S TIPS

Don't obsess. Your running shouldn't monopolize you while you're pregnant. If you need to stop running, it won't take that long to start up again after the baby is born.

Make running a constant. When everything is changing with pregnancy, running can be the one thing you count on. Get yourself out there, and you'll feel good the whole day after your run.

Your baby might fall asleep during your runs in the early months, and as she gets older, she actually may become bored. Books and small toys will help, but keep an eye on her. After all, what could be more fun than flinging something from the stroller and watching Mommy dive for it? Talk to her and point out the interesting sights. Your runs can be more than just exercise for you; they provide time for the two of you to bond and for her to learn new things.

Building a Babysitting Network

Sooner or later you'll probably need a babysitter so you can run consistently or to take care of the other aspects of your busy life. To find and keep the good ones, you have to be creative, resourceful, and flexible. Cast a wide net. Get to know your neighbors' teens and preteens and find out if they sit. If your child attends day care while you work, ask the teachers if they moonlight. Ask around at your place of worship or social club. Be open to unexpected opportunities and don't be timid. It never hurts to ask.

My friend Melissa David, a runner and mother of three from Winnetka, Illinois, suggests, "Look in unexpected places, not just the high school girl next door. Our cleaning lady is now sitting for us. And at our church we met a college student working on a degree in early childhood education. She's sitting for us now, too."

Screen sitters carefully, even if they come highly recommended. Look for a basic sense of respect. Does she appear to respect herself, and does she treat you with respect? How does she speak about the people in her life? Self-confidence is another deciding factor. Once you've trained her, will she be comfortable making the small decisions that crop up? Does she use common sense? If there is a fire in your house, you want someone who will grab your baby and run to safety. Does she love children in general and your child in particular? Watch how your child responds to her (when she's old enough to respond); her actions will tell you everything.

The more names on your roster, the better. Adult sitters usually have "real" jobs and other complications that may interfere with watching your child. Teenage babysitters often have school activities that will vary from month to month or semester to semester. Sometimes their babysitting job ranks last after schoolwork, sports, and special activities.

Once you find babysitters you like, you need to keep them interested. Find out what the going rate is for babysitting in your region, then pay at the higher end if you can afford to. Leave a little room for a raise, and give it to her within 3 to 6 months if she proves herself. Give kudos when she takes initiative, shows creativity, or does something special for your child. Tip generously for "extras" if you can. Find out if you can help her reach some of her goals. For example, offer yourself as a reference for future job applications.

Provide her with a list—spoken or written, depending on her style— of ways she can comfort and entertain your child. Update the list as your child gets older. Keep the baby's things organized and easy to find to make the sitter's job less complicated. Ask what else you can do to make her job easier. Make clear what you expect from her. If you don't want the TV on, tell her. Gently correct any behavior you don't like and guide her in the right direction, but also respect her style of care, even if it differs a little from yours.

A few simple actions will give your sitter confidence and provide you with peace of mind as you head out the door. Confirm that she knows what to do in case of emergency. If she's young, designate a neighbor she can contact, and double-check that the neighbor is home. Write down your cell phone number next to your home phone and carry the cell phone with you.

Preparing to Run through Another Pregnancy

Someday you may want another baby and you may want to run during that pregnancy, too. What can you do about it now? First, start working on your weaknesses. What was hard for you during this pregnancy? If your back was perpetually sore, try building strength in your abdominal and back muscles. If your knees hurt, strengthen the muscles in your legs that support your knees.

Studies show that it takes a woman's body about 18 months to restore nutrient levels after a pregnancy, so it's ideal to put at least that much time between the birth of one baby and the conception of the next. Continue taking a multivitamin with folic acid and zinc in case the stork comes early.

A FINAL NOTE

Motherhood places heavy claims on your energy—physical, emotional, and mental. You can become consumed by how well your baby is developing, whether she is getting sick, and whether either of you will sleep tonight. If you work outside the home, your energy drains even further.

Running gives you energy. It creates a quiet space between all the demands—it's a time to appreciate the quiet rhythm of your body at work, to unearth the person you've always been and to celebrate her. Moms who run find plenty to motivate them. It doesn't matter whether you focus on time splits or jog to enjoy the scenery. You might solve one important problem or contemplate hundreds of ideas.

Your prenatal running provided a bridge between your running life before children and your running life as a mother. Turn around and look back over your bridge. Reminisce a little and feel proud. Running during your pregnancy was an accomplishment, a true test of strength and endurance. Savor the experience because soon enough it will fade in your memory. Like your first mile and your first road race, your prenatal running will become part of your running history.

RESOURCE GUIDE

BOOKS

The Complete Book of Running for Women by Claire Kowalchik
Simon & Schuster, 1999

Exercising Through Your Pregnancy by James F. Clapp III, M.D.
Addicus Books, 2002

Maternal Fitness by Julie Tupler, R.N., with Andrea Thompson
Fireside, 1996

Nancy Clark's Sports Nutrition Guidebook by Nancy Clark, R.D.Human Kinetics, 1997

Pre- and Post-Natal Fitness by Lenita Anthony
American Council on Exercise, 2002

Pregnancy Fitness by the editors of *Fitness* magazine with Ginny Graves
Three Rivers Press, 1999

Runner's World Complete Book of Women's Running by Dagny Scott
Rodale, 2002

What to Expect When You're Expecting by Arlene Eisenberg, Heidi E. Murkoff, and Sandee E. Hathaway, B.S.N.
Workman Publishing, 2002

WEB SITES

American College of Obstetricians and Gynecologists
www.acog.com

***Fit Pregnancy* magazine**
www.fitpregnancy.com

LifeMatters
E-zine with articles and links on parenting, health, fitness, and nutrition
www.lifematters.com

March of Dimes
www.modimes.org

Melpomene Institute
Organization that researches and publishes information on women's health and fitness
www.melpomene.org

National Institutes of Health
www.nih.gov

***Runner's World* magazine**
www.runnersworld.com

***Runner's World* women's running**
www.womens-running.com

WORKOUT CLOTHING AND ACCESSORIES

Athleta Sports
Sells a limited variety of Mothers in Motion and InSport maternity workout clothes. (Use this site to compare prices.)
(888) 322-5515
www.athleta.com

Fit Maternity and Beyond
Thorough collection of workout clothing for pregnant athletes, along with pertinent books, videos, and "pregnancy comfort items"
(888) 961-9100
www.fitmaternity.com

InSport athletic apparel
Limited selection of maternity workout wear
(800) 652-5200
www.insport.com

Mothers in Motion
Complete line of workout clothing for pregnant athletes
(877) 512-8800
www.mothers-in-motion.com

Nike
Nike has teamed with maternity clothes designer Liz Lange to produce a stylish line of maternity workout gear.
www.niketown.com or
www.lizlange.com

Prenatal Cradle, Inc.
Doctor-recommended support garment for pregnant women who exercise
www.prenatalcradle.com

Road Runner Sports
Limited selection of maternity clothes, but excellent variety of running bras and other gear
(800) 636-3560
www.roadrunnersports.com

Title 9 Sports
Limited selection of maternity workout wear
(800) 609-0092
www.title9sports.com

INDEX

Underscored page references indicate boxed text. **Boldface** references indicate photographs.

Cooldown, 80, 89
Corset bra, <u>185</u>
Cosmetic changes, 162
   skin discolorations, 162
   spider veins, 163–64
   stretch marks, 162
   varicose veins, 162–63
Cough syrup, 106
Cranberry juice, 106
Cross-country runners, 29
Cross-country skiing, 59–60
Cross-country ski machines, 61
Cross-training, 10, 35
   cross-country skiing, 59–60
   cycling, 58–59
   deep-water running, <u>54</u>, 55
   exercise machines, 60–61
   group exercise classes, 56–58, 59
   Pilates, 61–62
   swimming, 53–54
   walking, 56
   water aerobics, <u>54</u>, 54–55
Crunch exercise, **13**
C-section. *See* Cesarean section
Curl-up (partial situp), **12**
   with a twist, **16**
Cycling fitness, 10, 58–59

D

Dads-to-be, 101
Dairy products, 74
Dead bug exercise, **14**
Decongestants, 106
Deep venous thrombosis, <u>128–29</u>
Deep-water running, <u>54</u>, 55
Dehydration, 93, 106
Delivery, 188–89. *See also* Labor and
   delivery
Depression, postpartum, 194–96
Dessert
   healthy, 74
   menu, 67, 68, 69, 70, 71, 72
Diabetes, gestational, 4, <u>126–27</u>,
   152–53, 170
Diarrhea, 182
Diastasis recti, <u>163</u>

Diet. *See* Nutritional needs
Dietary fat, 27, 32, 64, 204
Dinner menu, 67, 68, 69, 70, 71
Dizziness, 80, <u>99</u>, 104, 135–36
Dogs, avoiding threatening, <u>137</u>
Downhill skiing, warning about, <u>58</u>
Dumbbells, **46**, 55

E

Early-pregnancy mistakes, 79
Eating disorders, 29–33
Eating habits. *See* Nutritional needs
Eclampsia, 152, 171
Edema, 151–52
Eighth month, pregnancy symptoms
   during, 167–68
   feelings and sensations, 168–69
   your concerns, 169–73, 176–77
Elliptical trainers, 61
Embryo development, 77
Emergency deliveries, 170, 189. *See*
   also Labor and delivery
Emotional changes, during
   eighth month, 168–69
   fifth month, 131–35
   first month, 78–80
   fourth month, 118–19, 122–23
   recovery after delivery, 193–94
   second month, 92–95
   seventh month, 158–59
   sixth month, 144–47, 150–51
   third month, 103–6
Endorphins, 92, 114, <u>146</u>, 169, 171
Energy levels, 131–33, 136, 210
Energy sources, 8, 65
Engorgement pain, 205
Epidural, 165, 188, 190
Episiotomy incision, 173, 176, 188,
   <u>189</u>, 197
Estrogen, 27, 95, 125
Exercise
   fertility and, 26–27
   during pregnancy
      benefits of, 57–58, 147, <u>149</u>
      excessive, 26–27
      heart rate during, 81

Goals, personal, 150, 158–59, <u>159</u>, <u>161</u>
Grapevine motion exercise, **39**, 80
Grocery list, 72–74
Group exercise classes, 56–58, 59
Guilt, sense of, 158–59

H

Hamstrings
  strengthening exercise for, **45**, **52**
  stretching exercise for, **42**
Hang gliding, warning about, <u>58</u>
Heartburn, 54, 133–34, 159
Heart rate, monitoring, 6, 81, <u>88</u>, <u>121</u>
High blood pressure, <u>99</u>, <u>126–27</u>, 152. *See also* Hypertension, pregnancy-induced
High-impact aerobics, 57–58
High-risk pregnancy, 102
Hiking, 56
Hip muscles, strengthening exercise for, **45**, **52**, 59, 110
Hip problems, 111
Hitting the wall, <u>159</u>
Horseback riding, warning about, <u>58</u>
Hospital bag, 176
Humor, sense of, 7
Hydration levels, monitoring, 8, 65, 87, 89, 100, 151, 171–73, 204
Hyperemesis gravidarum, 93
Hypertension, pregnancy-induced, 102, <u>126–27</u>, 152, 170. *See also* High blood pressure
Hypothermia, 86–87

I

Ibuprofen, <u>80</u>, 110
Ice packs, 192–93
Identification card, 136
Illness prevention, 106–7. *See also* Pregnancy problems
Immune system function, 106–7

Incisions, vaginal, 170, 173, 176, 188, 197
Incompetent cervix, 99
Incontinence, urinary, 105–6, 144, 171, 202, <u>203</u>
Indoor tracks, 86
Induced labor, 183
Infertility specialist, 5, 26, <u>26</u>, 31, 78
Injury risks, 9–10, <u>22</u>, 107, 110, 147
Intelligence, of children born to exercising mothers-to-be, 4
Iron intake, 7, 9, 124, 125
Itchy skin, 133

J

Jogging exercise, 80, 87, <u>88</u>, 89
Joints and ligaments, 9, <u>22</u>, 35, 55, 95
Journal, running, <u>79</u>, 150
Juices, fruit, 65, 74, 106, 124
Junk food addicts, 7

K

Kegel exercises, 23, 44, 106, 144–46, 202
Knee pain, 89, 119
Knees, stretching exercise for, **39**
Knock-kneed stance, <u>163</u>

L

Labor and delivery
  cesarean section, 167, 169–70, 189–90
  delivery procedures, 188–89
  early contractions, 123–24
  effect of prenatal running on, <u>181</u>
  false labor, 182–83
  fears about, 164–64
  induced labor, 183
  natural childbirth, 165, <u>189</u>
  real labor, 165, 183, 186–88
Lateral flexion crunch, **17**

Pre-pregnancy physical examination, 5

Pre-pregnancy preparation, guidelines for
assessing your situation, 5
finding a supportive doctor, 6
getting your body ready, 9–10
making good food choices, 7–9
mentally gearing up, 6–7

Pre-pregnancy strengthening exercises
back extensor movements, 18–21
back extension, **18–19**
quadruped, **20–21**
flexion movements, 11–13
crunch, **13**
curl-up (partial situp), **12**
pelvic tilt, **11**
lateral flexion movement, 17
lateral flexion crunch, **17**
rotation movements, 14–16
curl-up with a twist, **16**
dead bug, **14**
modified bicycle, **15**

Presentation, of baby in womb, 167
Preterm birth risks, 4, <u>99</u>, 102, 128
Progesterone, 95, 100, 123, 125
Protein intake, 8, 27, 31, 63, 64–65, 136, 204
Prune juice, 124
Pubic pain, 111
Pubic symphysis, 111
Pubococcygeal (PC) muscles, 23, 44, 144
Pushing stage of labor, 188
Pushup
"girl," **48**
yoga, **47**

Q

Quadriceps muscles
strengthening exercise for, **45**, 58, 60
stretching exercise for, **41**
Quadruped exercises, for
pregnancy, **50–51**
pre-pregnancy, **20–21**

R

Range of motion, 59, 62
Recovery, after delivery, 192–97, <u>193</u>
advice from running moms, 85, <u>109</u>, <u>121</u>, <u>139</u>, <u>149</u>, <u>161</u>, <u>175</u>, <u>185</u>, <u>195</u>, <u>207</u>
cesarean and, 169, 193, <u>201</u>
going home, 192
ice pack for, 192–93
postpartum depression and, 194–96
resting and walking, 196–97
your emotions and, 193–94
Rectal temperature, 83
Recumbent stationary bikes, 59
Relaxin hormone, 95, 107
Rest and relaxation, 92, 131–33, 196
Rewards, as running motivation, 151
RICE treatment, <u>80</u>, <u>112</u>
Rotation movements, for abdominal muscles, 14–16
curl-up with a twist, **16**
dead bug, **14**
modified bicycle, **15**
Round-ligament pain, 111
Routes, 9, 136, 150
RPE, 81, <u>82</u>, <u>88</u>, 89
Runner's knee, 110–11
Running bras, 83, 95, 119, 122, 134, <u>185</u>, 204
Running buddies, 58, <u>139</u>, 140–41, 151
Running clothes. *See* Clothing, workout
Running gait, changes in, 43, 110, 179
Running routes, 9, 136, 150
Running sensations, 9
Running shoes, 86, 89, <u>97</u>, <u>105</u>, 118–19

S

Safety guidelines, 113–14, 136–37, 140, 171
Saliva ovulation detector, <u>30</u>